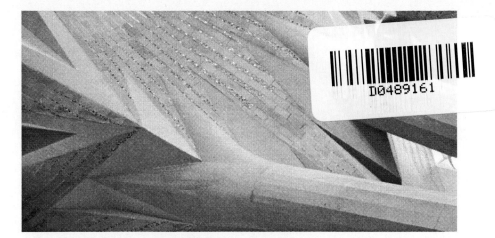

Effective Communication Skills for Doctors

A practical guide to clear communication within a hospital environment

Teresa Parrot & Graham Crook

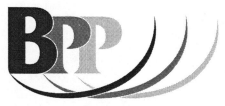

LEARNING MEDIA

First edition September 2011

ISBN 9781 4453 7956 2

British Library Cataloguing-in-Publication Data
A catalogue record for this book is available from
the British Library

Published by
BPP Learning Media Ltd
BPP House, Aldine Place
London W12 8AA

www.bpp.com/health

Typeset by Replika Press Pvt Ltd, India
Printed in the United Kingdom

Your learning materials, published by BPP
Learning Media Ltd, are printed on paper
sourced from sustainable, managed forests.

Contents

Contents

About the Publisher

BPP Learning Media is dedicated to supporting aspiring professionals with top quality learning material. BPP Learning Media's commitment to success is shown by our record of quality, innovation and market leadership in paper-based and e-learning materials. BPP Learning Media's study materials are written by professionally-qualified specialists who know from personal experience the importance of top quality materials for success.

Free Companion Material

Readers can access a free online module and download a certificate of completion to strengthen their learning/revalidation/CPD portfolio.

To access the above companion material please visit **www.bbp.com/freehealthresources**

About the Authors

Dr Teresa Parrott BM MRCPsych MSc

Teresa graduated in medicine from Southampton University in 1987. She trained in Psychiatry and became a member of the Royal College of Psychiatrists in 1992. She worked for two years in medium secure units, and completed an MSc in Forensic Mental Health at St George's in 2008. She saw patients for psychodynamic psychotherapy for four years under supervision. She attended an Experiential Analytical Group and has undergone personal analytical psychotherapy. She currently works as a consultant psychiatrist in Scotland.

Dr Graham Crook MB ChB MRCP

Graham qualified in medicine from Aberdeen University in 1979. He spent two years of his post-graduate training at the Royal Brompton Hospital in London and became a Consultant in General Medicine (1988) and Chest Medicine (1990). He was Officer Commanding the RAF Chest Unit from 1989 until 1993 and was Consultant Adviser in Chest Medicine to the Director General Medical Services (RAF). He left the RAF in 1993 and moved to Spain. He has always enjoyed teaching including MRCP, Respiratory Medicine and Aviation Medicine courses. He runs workshops in personal development and meditation.

Acknowledgements

Teresa Parrott and Graham Crook are indebted to Helen Hayward, MBBS, MRCP, who co-authored Chapter 9 'Life and death' of this book.

Dedications

To Peter
Teresa

To Catriona
Graham

Foreword

A quiet revolution has been taking place in the field of medical practice. Some practitioners have embraced the change and some, it seems, are unaware of its existence. This book charts the progress of the change, the reasons for the need for change, and gives much needed education and practical advice on how to get there. It is a must read, in my view, for all doctors and other health practitioners who are operating at the doctor/patient interface. I would also highly recommend it as an addition to reading lists for medical and nursing training.

This book is about the relationship between doctor and patient, and the communication (or lack thereof) between them. The goal of the book is to 'help doctors to improve the ways that they interact – with patients, with other doctors, and ultimately with themselves.' Parrott and Crook show how the traditional stance of the doctor, as the paternalistic and powerful authority figure in relation to the patient as needy supplicant to be done to, has become outdated. The balance of power has shifted. They describe how healthcare is increasingly becoming a partnership. The emphasis has moved from a doctor-centred or disease-centred model to a patient-centred model, in which the patient is much more involved in decisions. In this context the traditional biomedical approach is not enough because it does not take adequate account of the psychological and social factors which are now recognised as being crucial in the understanding of illness development, treatment and recovery.

The NHS has changed, and patients are now regarded as consumers with choices, who have rights and access to information, expectations that they will be listened to, communicated with and have the opportunity to take an active part in their treatment programme. Therefore, doctors now need to have the communication skills and a range of psychological know-how in order to work with their patients in a more holistic way. In a carefully researched and highly readable book, Parrott and Crook show how this can be achieved. They invite the medical profession to move on by 'finding new ways of interacting that work better than the old, using communication as a bridge – between insight and action, between the wisdom of the past and the vision of the future.'

In twelve chapters they cover how doctors communicate, communication theory, communication skills, and how to improve communication. They then look at more practical issues including different models for the medical interview, barriers to communication, issues about life and death, how to break bad news, and how to deal with difficult situations. Interspersed within this is also discussion of the importance of the holistic approach and how the doctor patient relationship in and of itself can provide a healing framework. Finally they talk about the continuing importance of personal development and self support throughout the career cycle. Parrott and Crook are advocating a humane blend of information sharing, empathic understanding and therapeutic exchange to stand alongside of traditional biomedical practice. In case this sounds new age and woolly, at every stage, they present the scientific research which shows a strong evidence base for what they are advocating. This is a gem of a book and I cannot do justice to the wealth of information that it contains.

The book begins with a traditional research orientated presentation of the facts; a suitable beginning since they are addressing themselves to a medical audience. But then they begin to infiltrate the facts with the occasional personal anecdote or case discussion. They are moving from the medical model to a more participatory, patient orientated perspective. The reader is being encouraged to take a more active role and to begin to empathise and feel, as well as think. Having introduced the idea of communication theory and communication skills, in Chapter 5 the authors take us into a discussion of how to improve communication and focus on the key issues of empathy, the development of rapport, the importance of the relationship and the idea of emotional intelligence. This is a very important chapter and it leads well into the next chapter which gives us a description of a number of different models of the medical interview, including the medical model, the biopsychosocial model, the psychodynamic model and the holistic model. What is so crucial here is that all models are relevant.

In Chapter 7 we have a consideration of some barriers to communication, including cultural and racial differences, power dynamics, attitudes (Weston & Lipkin, 1989: 'in would sweep twelve coats, never introduce themselves, discourse loudly over the bed in technical jargon and then sweep out without a word')

and time constraints. If you only have ten minutes per patient it is very hard to sit and listen and try and understand, without interrupting the patient and taking them in the direction you think they need to go. As Parrott and Crook point out, in this scenario, so much gets missed.

Chapter 8 talks about healing through the relationship. This chapter begins with a painful description of one woman's experience of the medical profession following the discovery of a breast lump. What is painful is not so much the lump itself, but the way in which she is treated. Parrott and Crook quote Bub (2006):

> *healing does not occur in isolation, it emerges from a healing relationship. Communication heals when it provides safety, support, relief of isolation, encourages re-telling of the trauma story, reflects back the best self of the individual, reminds the patient of his/her identity besides that of patient, and supports the processing and integration of emotion.*

The woman with the lump is treated like an object; other examples given in this chapter show how so much difference is made when the patient is respected as a human being.

The next chapter deals with how best to break bad news to the patient, and the authors give some useful summaries of things that need to be borne in mind by the doctor in this kind of situation. Breaking bad news is painful and difficult for both patient and doctor, and finding ways to take care of both, seems really important. Lots of examples of good and bad practice in this chapter, and also a consideration of how to help the doctor to cope with grief – their own and that of other members of the team, patients and their relatives. A complex and distressing issue which needs to be given thought and time. In Chapter 10 the authors talk about other difficult situations and give some helpful advice on how to manage aggressive and violent patients, including methods of de-escalation. Chapter 11 is concerned with support, supervision and personal development – vital issues which all too often get overlooked in an ordinary busy practice setting. The changes in attitudes to patients which are portrayed so well in this book, go alongside of a necessary re-evaluation of doctors' own attitudes towards themselves. Taking care must occur in every direction.

Finally, in Chapter 12 Parrott and Crook provide a useful summary of key learning points in the book. I am a psychotherapist, and I have always therefore seen the importance of communication. But in my relationships with the medical profession over 60 years, as a patient, as a therapist working in a hospital setting and as a relative of a patient, I have experienced many examples of non-existent, poor, sometimes appalling communication. And I am not unique. This book is needed.

Dr Eva Coleman
Psychoanalytic Psychotherapist

Chapter 1
Introduction

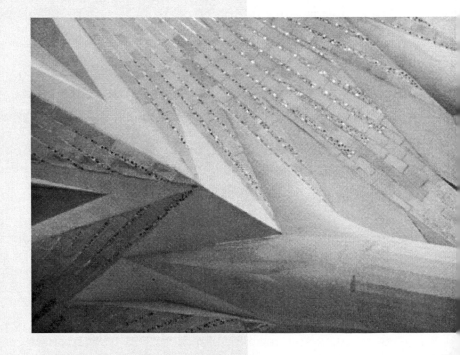

Introduction

The last fifteen years have seen unprecedented changes in medicine and the role of doctors. Communication skills are essential to these new roles.

This book attempts a synthesis of the most important theories and research in the field of communication. And more specifically in the field of doctor-patient interaction. There is a large and compelling evidence base which shows not only that communication is vitally important to both doctors and patients, but that changes are necessary in the attitudes and skills that underlie the way that doctors communicate.

This book aims to explain the factors driving change. Once we can understand why change is necessary, it becomes easier to accept. The book also explores what tools are needed to help facilitate the changes required.

The overall goal is to show that, by fine-tuning their communication skills, doctors can improve their personal efficacy and enhance their relationships with patients, with other doctors – and ultimately with themselves.

Why do doctors need to communicate better?

90% of the public are satisfied with the way doctors do their jobs, 96% are satisfied with the way nurses do their jobs (NHS Plan 2000). A MORI poll in 2009 revealed that 92% of the public said they trusted doctors to tell the truth. However, there is growing evidence that patients are complaining about poor communication with their doctors.

The Picker Institute Europe found that almost half of hospital inpatients and a third of patients consulting their general practitioners would have liked more involvement in decisions about their care (RCP, 2005).

The Healthcare Commission reported that about a third of patients they surveyed received conflicting information from health professionals; sometimes the information given about diagnostic

2

tests, possible treatment side-effects, and discharge medications was confused or non-existent (Healthcare Commission, 2005).

The Bristol Inquiry (2001) recommended that patients must be at the centre of the NHS and must be treated as partners by health professionals – as 'equals with different expertise' (Coulter, 2002). However, reports of research by Coulter (2001) from the *Expert Patient* (DH, 2001b) describe some common experiences of patients:

- Not enough involvement in decisions.
- No-one to talk to about anxieties and concerns.
- Tests and/or treatments not clearly explained.
- Insufficient information for family/friends.
- Insufficient information about recovery.

The Centre for Change and Innovation (2003) reports that the Lothian Hospitals NHS Trust asked patients for their views:

> *60% complained about a lack of involvement in decisions about their care*
> *33% said they had been given no explanation of test results*
> *31% said they had no opportunity to talk to the doctor*
> *23% complained of nurses and doctors saying different things.*
> (BMA, 2004)

Communication difficulties are one of the main reasons that patients complain about doctors. The most common criticism is not about the doctor's competence but rather that he or she has failed either to listen or to offer sufficient explanation (RCP, 1997). According to the British Medical Association (BMA, 2004), patients are less likely to complain or to sue if doctors communicate well. Reports from the medical defence societies, the Health Service Ombudsman, and serious incident enquiries all point to the need for better communication (RCP, 1997).

Lack of adequate communication skills also has important implications for the mental health of doctors (RCP, 1997). Problematic communication with patients is thought to contribute to emotional burnout and low personal accomplishment in doctors as well as high psychological morbidity (Feinman, 2002). Ramirez *et al.* (1996) reported that burnout among consultants was associated with low satisfaction with relationships with patients, relatives and staff, and was more prevalent in those who felt insufficiently trained in communication and management skills.

How the role of doctors is changing

The last two decades have seen unprecedented changes in medicine. These changes have been happening at all levels, from government directives to patient expectations.

The National Health Service (NHS) has been reformed, with new direction, structure and management. The demographics of diseases and of the population itself are changing: people are living longer, disease patterns are shifting, and there are more chronic illnesses. The biomedical model, in which doctors have traditionally been trained, does not take adequate account of psychological and social factors which are not only relevant to chronic illness, but also are of increasing importance in the management of those rising numbers of patients for whom there is no medical diagnosis or physical explanation of symptoms.

Health care is increasingly a partnership. The emphasis has shifted from a doctor-centred or disease-centred model to a patient-centred model, in which the patient is now much more involved in decisions. Patient expectations are changing. Patients are increasingly seen as consumers of health care; they have rights defined within the NHS Constitution, and they are better informed as a result of a much wider range of health information available through the Internet and other sources. There is a new emphasis on prevention of illness and health promotion.

These changes have all had a profound effect on the role of doctors.

Doctors have been trained to do certain tasks extremely well. The vast majority of doctors work hard to do their best for their patients. However, within the last decade, they have been asked to fulfil additional roles and to take on new responsibilities. The model that they have been taught does not very well suit the tasks with which they are now faced, and it omits certain aspects, previously not seen as important, that have now become essential.

Communication skills are vital to these new roles. They form the basis of new relationships with patients, of the development of the partnership approach, of new styles of interaction with managers, colleagues and other members of the team. Doctors are now expected to participate in management and leadership at all levels of their training and career, and this requires a different style of communication.

The changing NHS

The government White Paper *The NHS Plan* (2000) announced new investment in health, and heralded the beginning of a ten-year redirection of the NHS. Major issues emerging from public consultation were that people wanted more staff, shorter waiting times, and care centred on patients. People frequently felt that they were not listened to, and in-patient satisfaction with hospital care had been decreasing since 1989 (Mercer *et al.*, 2001), to the point that 10 to 20% of patients were dissatisfied across the country.

In response to this apparently widespread public dissatisfaction with healthcare services, it was decided that the NHS would be redesigned to become patient-centred. This meant, as outlined in the core principles of the Plan, that patients would be treated as individuals; that partnerships would develop between patients and staff; and that patients would have more say in their own treatment.

The Plan stated that 'By 2002, it will be a pre-condition of qualification to deliver patient care in the NHS that an individual has demonstrated competence in communication with patients.' In addition, 'all doctors will, as a condition of contract, be required to participate in annual appraisal, and clinical audit, from 2001.'

The Department of Health (DH) document *Working Together* (2001a) suggested further reasons for the accelerating changes in healthcare, including:

- Increased availability of research-based knowledge.
- The rise of empowered, knowledgeable consumers.
- The re-shaping of processes and pathways to support care that is truly patient-centred.

- A greater emphasis on team working.
- An emphasis on ease of patient access to services (NHS Direct, one stop 'walk-in' centres).

The Darzi Report in June 2008 outlined the particular difficulties faced by the NHS in this century, which included: rising expectations; demand driven by demographics; the continuing development of the 'information society;' and the changing nature of disease. It also stated the extent of the investment in the NHS. Since the NHS Plan in 2000, there had been an increase in the NHS budget for England from £33 billion in 1996/7 to £96 billion in 2008/9, with 5,000 more GPs employed and 33,000 more hospital doctors.

In 2009, however, the financial situation changed due to the global recession. Following this period of expansion, the NHS was faced with far-reaching budgetary cuts.

In addition, the introduction of the European Working Time Directive has made a substantial impact on doctors' training and working lives. A survey of junior doctors by the Royal College of Surgeons (RCS) in 2005 showed that – since implementation of the directive – 75% of juniors think that continuity of care has deteriorated, around 90% think that direct contact with patients and training have decreased, and more than half of specialist registrars think that their quality of life is worse on partial shifts (Lowry & Cripps, 2005). Ahmed-Little (2009) states that the reduction from 56 to 48 hours a week will lead to 'another 12% fall in daytime availability of junior doctors in the average rotation, further decreasing direct contact with patients, quality of care, and training of junior staff.'

Changes in demographics

In most developed countries, people are living longer, and as a result, disease patterns are changing. There are more chronic or long-term illnesses such as heart disease, stroke, cancer, arthritis, diabetes, mental illness, asthma and other conditions (*Expert Patient*, DH, 2001b).

In the UK, as many as 17.5 million adults suffer from a chronic disease – at least one person in three, rising to 75% of those aged 75 or more (*Expert Patient*, DH 2001b). Six million people care for family or friends with chronic illness.

Mental health problems have become much more prevalent: they are now the most frequent causes of sick leave (Confederation of British Industry, 2005); they account for at least one in four GP consultations (NHS Plan, 2000), and it is estimated that they affect up to 20% of the child and adolescent population (*Expert Patient*, DH 2001b).

Medically unexplained symptoms, which are physical symptoms which have no medical diagnosis or explanation, are also increasing in prevalence. They account for a considerable proportion of consultations by frequent attenders in secondary care (Reid *et al.*, 2001). For example, Hamilton *et al.* (1996) reported rates of medically unexplained symptoms of 53%, 42%, and 32% in gastroenterology, neurology, and cardiology respectively; this finding was confirmed by Nimnuan *et al.* (2000), who looked at seven specialist clinics in one hospital and found that 51% of new patients were diagnosed as having medically unexplained symptoms (Reid *et al.*, 2001).

At the Citizens' Summit in Birmingham in 2005, which was part of the public consultation process for the DH White Paper in 2006 (Our health, our care, our say), 75% of people said that they wanted a regular health check or MOT for everyone; 63% wanted a focus on mental well-being, and 42% wanted more help for carers.

The NHS Constitution, published by the Department of Health in January 2009, sets out the principles and values of the NHS, including a commitment to high-quality care that is safe, effective and focused on patient experience. 'NHS services must reflect the needs and preferences of patients, their families and carers. Patients, with their families and carers, where appropriate, will be involved in and consulted on all decisions about their care and treatment.'

The Constitution reflects a changing ethos within healthcare provision. It states quite clearly that patients must participate in all decisions about treatment. In other words, the doctor is no longer expected to weigh the balance alone.

In order to make these choices, patients must be offered 'easily accessible, reliable and relevant information.' It is not enough that the doctor is informed; it is his responsibility also to communicate this information to the patient, who has 'the right to be involved in discussions and decisions about healthcare' (DH, 2009).

Traditional communication skills training

In the past, communication skills training was not an integral part of medical education. In traditional medical training, medical interviewing was doctor-centred; the biomedical model formed the foundation of the doctor's approach, and the doctor's role was confined to diagnosis of disease, management and treatment. There was simply no mention of a patient-centred or holistic approach.

The disadvantages of traditional medical training have been widely described in the literature:

- It is not correct to assume that doctors either have the ability to communicate empathically with their patients or that they will acquire this ability during their medical training (Sanson-Fisher & Poole, 1978 in Kurtz *et al.*, 2005).
- A well known study of medical education found that medical students' interpersonal skills with patients declined as their medical education progressed (Helfer, 1970 in Roter & Hall, 2006).
- Without specific training in communication skills, medical students' ability to communicate deteriorates as they progress through their traditional medical training. They enter medical school with better communication skills than when they leave (Kurtz *et al.*, 2005).
- Traditionally, a medical approach to history-taking, based on the belief that every illness is caused by a disease with an external definable cause, has predominated. Taking a history in this formal and structured way tends to make consultations disease or doctor-centred (Thistlethwaite & Jordan, 1999).
- Unfortunately, although traditional methods of medical education are good at teaching young doctors their purely clinical skills, the acquisition of any effective consulting style has tended to be arbitrary and fortuitous (Neighbour, 2005).
- Often established doctors can remember few times in the whole of their medical training when they were directly observed interacting with patients (Kurtz *et al.*, 2005).

- In essence medical history-taking means collecting answers to our well-tried set of questions. More often than not practically everything else that the patient tries to tell his doctor is pushed aside as irrelevant (Balint, 1957).
- Paternalism is widely regarded as the traditional form of the doctor-patient relationship and it is still seen as the most common one (Emanuel & Emanuel, 1992 in Roter & Hall, 2006).
- Roter & Hall (2006) state that: 'indications are that medical students are affected by training and that their attitudes change as they progress through medical school – they become more negative. Medical students become less patient-centred and more paternalistic in their attitudes (Haidet *et al.*, 2002), less favourably disposed towards providing care to medically indigent patients (Crandall *et al.*, 1993), less idealistic and less positive in regard to the elderly and patients in chronic pain (Griffith & Wilson, 2001), and less inclined to believe in the importance of discussing psychosocial concerns (Williams & Deci, 1996).'
- Salinsky & Sackin (2000) quote McWhinney (1999) who states that 'Western medicine, at least for the past 100 years, has neglected the emotions.' Their view is that 'the emotional education of doctors has to be one of the basic themes of the educational process, informing everything else.'
- Thistlethwaite & Jordan (1999) report that students are rarely exposed to the concept of patient-centred consultations during ward-based teaching. They are less likely to observe doctors asking about patients' concerns during teaching sessions in hospital. There is also a lack of encouragement to delve into a patient's social history which may have a bearing on the patient's problems and subsequent outcome.
- Many experienced physicians have good communication skills, but changing the working practices of those who lack them is likely to be difficult. Even those who communicate well may not be aware of the best ways to teach communication skills to their trainees, although heavy reliance may be placed on them to provide this aspect of training (RCP, 1997).

The patient-centred approach

There are various definitions of patient-centred care. Stewart (2001) states that patients want patient-centred care which:

- Explores the patient's main reason for the visit, concerns, and need for information;
- Seeks an integrated understanding of the patients' world – that is, their whole person, emotional needs, and life issues;
- Finds common ground on what the problem is and mutually agrees on management; enhances prevention and health promotion;
- Enhances the continuing relationship between the patient and the doctor.

The Institute of Medicine (2001) defines patient-centred care as: 'Health care that establishes a partnership among practitioners, patients, and their families (when appropriate) to ensure that decisions respect patients' wants, needs, and preferences, and that patients have the education and support they need to make decisions and participate in their own care.'

Little *et al.* (2001a) identified three groupings of patient preferences:

- Communication: including listening, exploration of concerns, and requirements for information, doctor-patient relationship and a clear explanation;
- Partnership: including specific aspects of communication related to finding common ground, such as exploration, discussion, and mutual agreement about patients' ideas, the problem, and treatment;
- Health promotion: including how to stay healthy and reduce the risk of future illness.

The more holistic, patient-centred approach recognises that a problem may be defined in terms of its physical, psychological and/or social components. Not only does the doctor need to be aware of the nature and cause of the problem, but also s/he should investigate the patient's ideas, concerns and expectations as part of the management process (Thistlethwaite & Jordan, 1999).

The patient-centred method aims not only to diagnose the patient's disease but also to understand the meaning of the illness for the patient (McWhinney, 1989).

Holman & Lorig (2000) make the point that when acute disease was the primary cause of illness, patients were generally inexperienced and passive recipients of medical care. Now that chronic disease has become the principal medical problem, the patient must become a co-partner in the process. The DH document *Trust, Assurance and Safety* (2007) reinforces the idea of the health professional and patient entering into an open, honest and active partnership. The *Expert Patient* (DH, 2001b) also states that a new relationship must be built in which health professionals and patients are genuine partners seeking together the best solutions to each patient's problem.

The new role of doctors

In 1981 only 30% of medical schools in the UK gave any teaching in communication skills (RCP, 1997). However, in 1993, the General Medical Council (GMC) emphasised the importance of the development of skills to interact with patients and colleagues (*Tomorrow's Doctors*, 1993), and many medical schools began to revise their teaching and assessment of communication skills (BMA, 2004).

Ten years later, *Tomorrow's Doctors* (2003) reinforced that graduates must be able to communicate clearly, sensitively and effectively with patients, relatives, and colleagues. The Quality Assurance Agency (QAA) was set up, which, in collaboration with the GMC, ensures that these interpersonal skills are being taught effectively within the medical curriculum. *Tomorrow's Doctors* (2003) also stipulated that graduates must be aware of current developments and guiding principles in the NHS, for example, patient-centred care, and the importance of working as a team within a multi-professional environment.

In 2004, the King's Fund produced a report (Rosen & Dewar, 2004) aiming to redefine the meaning of medical professionalism for better patient care. It stated that the traditional image of the professional was outdated, and that doctors should change tack, by defining a new 'compact' between themselves, government, the public, health-service managers, and patient groups, and by strengthening medical leadership.

In 2005, the Royal College of Physicians (RCP) set up a Working Party whose report offered a new definition of medical professionalism as:

> *A set of values, behaviours, and relationships that underpins the trust the public has in doctors. Medicine is a vocation in which a doctor's knowledge, clinical skills, and judgement are put in the service of protecting and restoring human well being. This purpose is realised through a partnership between patient and doctor, one based on mutual respect, individual responsibility, and appropriate accountability.*
>
> (RCP, 2005)

The report drew attention to the fact that the medical profession has been slow to adapt to changing societal expectations: management and leadership are for many doctors neglected areas. It stated that the interaction between doctor and manager is central to the delivery of professional care, and that a doctor's corporate responsibility, shared with managers and others, is a frequently neglected aspect of modern practice (RCP, 2005). Indeed, according to the BMA (2004), communication difficulties between doctors and managers are a leading cause of disciplinary problems.

The RCP report (2005) pointed out that many of the qualities of professionalism are not covered in the undergraduate medical curriculum or in postgraduate training. Doctors were often seen as poor communicators; arrogant, negative, defensive and self-serving, although they themselves believed that they had become much better at communicating with patients. For these reasons, the report recommended that doctors reflect on medical professionalism, and that the GMC should revise *Tomorrow's Doctors* (2003) to strengthen leadership and managerial skills as key competencies of professional practice. *Tomorrow's Doctors* (2009) has now been published, and medical schools are preparing for its application from 2011/12 onwards.

In 2006, the GMC revised *Good Medical Practice* (first published 1995), which set the standards for doctors at both undergraduate and postgraduate levels. It stated the need for a good working relationship with patients, based on trust, openness and good communication (GMC, 2006). *Good Medical Practice* defined effective communication as: listening to patients; respecting their views about their health; responding to their concerns and preferences; sharing information in ways that they can understand; and explaining the treatment options available, including associated risks and uncertainties.

In *The New Doctor* (2007), the GMC stated that in order to become fully registered, doctors must be able to:

> *Establish and maintain effective relationships with patients; encourage and support the patient to share all relevant information; recognise that patients are knowledgeable about themselves and the effect their health has on their daily life; encourage and support patients to be involved in their own care; and be sensitive to the needs and expectations of patients, taking into account their lifestyle, culture, religion, beliefs, ethnic background, sex, sexuality, disability, age or social or economic status.*

Communication skills are now regarded as a core competence. Assessment of communication skills will be necessary as part of the doctor's appraisal and personal development plans (BMA, 2004). The Postgraduate Medical Education Training Board (PMETB) has developed training curricula with all specialties, based on Good Medical Practice. The Royal Colleges now include communication skills' assessment in their training: the Royal College of General Practitioners (RCGP) are using video recordings for assessing communication skills in candidates, and the Royal College of Physicians has introduced communication skills assessment into its training (BMA, 2004).

The Academy of Medical Royal Colleges is developing the standards for specialist re-certification and revalidation (GMC: *Operationalising Good Medical Practice*, 2007) and also, in conjunction with the NHS Institute for Innovation and Improvement, has developed the Medical Leadership Competency Framework (2008). This states that all doctors and medical students must be actively involved in the planning, delivery and transformation of health services. Clark & Armit (2008) state that 'introduction of this Framework will have a significant impact on how doctors are trained. To be deemed an effective and safe doctor in the future, competence in both clinical and wider non-clinical competences including management and leadership will be required.'

Specifically, the Framework encourages development of personal qualities that enhance relationships and interactions with patients and colleagues. Self-awareness is defined as knowing your own strengths and weaknesses. It involves realising the impact of your behaviour on others, and the influence of your own emotions and prejudices on your judgments and behaviour. The aim of increasing self-awareness is to be able to manage the impact of your emotions in your day-to-day practice – and to improve your relationships overall.

The Framework emphasises the importance of listening, empathising, and gaining trust. The aim is that doctors will learn to manage services, resources, people and performance. By learning how to communicate effectively with both individuals and groups, and by encouraging and respecting the contribution of others, they will be better leaders – and members – of the multiprofessional team. By listening to patients, they will understand better the problems that exist within services, and be more able to make changes to improve the system.

A new philosophy

It is clear that there has been a recent and profound change in the role of doctors. Patients, managers, the public, the government are all calling for better services, and for different services. Older doctors are no longer practising medicine in the way that they expected to; they were not trained to be teachers, leaders or managers, yet their contracts now demand them to be. Younger doctors are learning the theory of management and leadership, in amongst an already vast curriculum they can barely keep up with. Both are compelled, like it or not, to become a new type of doctor.

The reality is that the authority and autonomy of doctors has been challenged in an unprecedented way. Doctors are now observed, appraised, and rated on both clinical and, latterly, non-clinical skills. They have been expected to take on a gradually expanding range of non-clinical roles and responsibilities that their training has not prepared them for. The demands of the new system have thrown the defects of the old into sharp focus.

This has understandably led to problems. Change imposed from outside – or above – is often resisted and resented. Perceived criticism generally provokes antagonism and alienation. To attempt different methods of working without the required skills in place is counterproductive and ineffectual. Stress at work ultimately leads to worse, not better, patient care.

We know that doctors are increasingly stressed at work. In 1994 it was found that the estimated prevalence of psychiatric morbidity was 27% among consultants in five specialties: gastroenterology, radiology, surgical oncology, clinical oncology, and medical oncology (Ramirez et al., 1996). By 2002, in the same five specialties, it had risen to 32%, and the prevalence of emotional exhaustion had increased from 32% in 1994 to 41% in 2002. Multivariate analysis showed that increased job stress without increase in job satisfaction accounted for the decline in mental health (Taylor et al., 2005).

It has been noted that doctors have a very high incidence of alcoholism, depressive illness and chronic stress disorders (Tate, 2007), and, in the UK, the suicide rate for doctors is approximately twice the national average (Ramirez et al, 1996). In 2005, over three-quarters of consultant physicians planned to take early retirement – a loss of over 6,000 person-years of experienced work from the health service (RCP, 2006).

We should be appalled at these statistics. The fact is that we're ashamed to admit that doctors are struggling. As a profession, we do not find it easy to ask for help. Also, as a profession, we are fragmented. We are lacking in leadership. There is 'almost no coherence of vision on many important issues facing patient care across the Royal Colleges and Faculties' (RCP, 2005). It is our belief that there is an urgent need to improve doctors' communication skills – for the reasons stated above. And because research has shown that poor communication can contribute to burnout among consultants, patient dissatisfaction, lack of compliance and increased medico-legal problems. Improved communication skills could impact positively on all of these.

We do have to change. We have to adapt to a new definition of 'professionalism,' a changed concept of what it means to be a doctor. We have to become confident leaders, capable managers, knowledgeable about non-clinical fields, at ease with communication and management theory – and yet also retain our humanity.

This book will help to make some of these difficult transitions easier. Skills can be learned, once we acknowledge the need for them. We can become more articulate and cohesive as a profession, we can enjoy better relationships, and make working practice more satisfying. We can equip ourselves with a new armoury of attitudes and strategies.

This book will explore how to communicate naturally – which means being yourself – and effectively, which means being what you need to be to others. Learning about yourself in order to learn about other people. Recognising what it is about the way that some patients communicate that makes them difficult to manage, and the way that some colleagues communicate that makes them difficult to relate to. Finding new ways of interacting that work better than the old, using communication as a bridge – between insight and action, between the wisdom of the past and the vision of the future.

Chapter 2

How doctors communicate

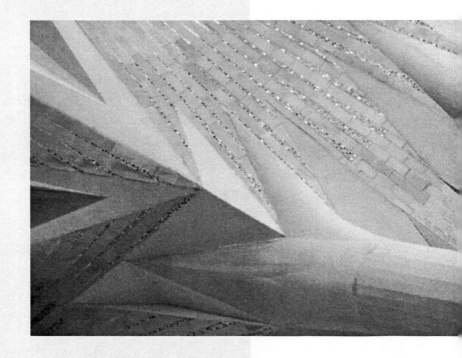

How doctors communicate

Introduction

Over the last fifty years a body of research investigating various aspects of doctor-patient communication has developed. This chapter presents what is known from the literature about how doctors actually communicate.

Background

As far back as 1951, there was evidence that doctors needed to be trained in how to communicate. Skills such as listening, expressing respect for patients, and awareness of nonverbal communication needed to be incorporated into medical practice. Korsch (1968) found that '24% of patients reported dissatisfaction, notably due to lack of warmth and friendliness on the part of the doctor, failure to take into account the patient's concerns and expectations, lack of clear-cut explanation, and use of medical jargon.' So poor communication is not a new problem.

In the UK in 1976, Byrne & Long analysed 2,500 patient visits, and published a paper which looked in depth for the first time at the way in which consultations in general practice were being conducted. They found that:

- Many doctors are not good listeners.
- The way in which a doctor sets about a consultation is largely repetitive.
- At least 20% of consultations show insensitivity on the part of the doctor.
- Many doctors feel hopeless when faced with a 'sick' patient who has nothing organic wrong with him.
- Few demonstrate the capacity to meet the needs of those patients whose problems do not fit into an organic disease pattern.

Byrne & Long distinguished between doctor-centred and patient-centred interviews, and emphasised the needs of the patient. They suggested that the doctor ought to find out what 'felt needs' had lead the patient to visit the doctor. This may seem obvious, but their work showed that in fact many doctors were having difficulties in discovering why the patient had come. They also found that few patients were being given the opportunity to be involved in their own treatment.

In 1979, Platt & McMath observed more than 300 clinical interviews and found that doctors were frequently inattentive to symptoms; they did not consider patient-centred data or active problems other than the present illness; they showed a high control style, and did not formulate needed working hypotheses.

In the US in 1984, Beckman & Frankel conducted a widely quoted study of 74 visits: 60 with internal medicine residents, and 14 with family practitioners. They found that:

- Doctors allowed patients to complete their opening statement in only 23% of visits.
- In 51 (69%) of the visits, the physician interrupted the patient's opening statement – after a mean time of only 18 seconds – and directed questions toward a specific concern.
- Once patients had been interrupted, they were unlikely to disclose further concerns.
- In only one of these 51 visits was the patient able to return to, and complete, their opening statement, ie the concerns for which they sought care.
- Given sufficient time and opportunity, the patient will mark the end of their opening statement of concerns.
- When allowed to finish, no patient's opening statement took more than 150 seconds.

Beckman *et al.* (1985) found that doctors were taking control of the content of the interview too early in the visit, and were choosing one problem to explore rather than eliciting the patient's full agenda, In addition, they found that patients who completed their statement of concerns in the opening moments of the encounter were significantly less likely to raise concerns toward the end of the visit (Frankel & Beckman, 1989).

In 1999, Marvel *et al.* repeated the original study to find out whether behaviour had changed. They conducted a study in the US and Canada of 29 family physicians. 264 visits were analysed; mean visit length was 15 minutes. Nine doctors had completed fellowship training in family therapy and communication skills. They found that:

- Only 28% of experienced physicians solicited the patient's complete agenda.
- The mean time available to patients to initially express their concerns before the first physician redirection was 23.1 seconds.
- Most redirections (76%) occurred after the first concern.
- Once the discussion became focused on a specific concern, the likelihood of returning to complete the agenda was very low. Patient concerns were eventually completed in only 8% of the visits.
- Patients who initiated one or more concerns and were given the opportunity to complete their concerns used an average of only 32 seconds.
- Physicians trained in family therapy and communication skills more frequently solicited concerns fully, often by an open-ended question followed by nondirective facilitating utterances (eg 'Uh-huh' or 'What else?') Having heard the patient's agenda, the multiple concerns were then explicitly prioritised with the patient.
- Using a simple opening solicitation, such as 'What concerns do you have?' then asking 'Anything else?' repeatedly until a complete agenda has been identified appears to take 6 seconds longer than interviews in which the patient's agenda is interrupted.

Langewitz *et al.* (1998, 2002) taught doctors to actively listen without interrupting, and examined how long it would take patients to indicate that they had completed their story—for example, with a statement such as: 'That's all, doctor!' Their study was conducted in an internal medicine outpatient clinic of a Swiss tertiary referral centre. Even with such complex patients, they found that:

- The mean spontaneous talking time was 92 seconds, and 78% (258) of patients had finished their initial statement in two minutes.
- Seven patients talked for longer than five minutes, but in all cases doctors felt that the patients were giving important information and should not be interrupted.

How do medical students rate on communication skills?

At the start of their medical training, students are 'alive with the prospect of helping people' (Shooter, 2002); they are good at using language appropriate to the patient, allowing patients to tell their own story, and using open-ended questions (Preven *et al.*, 1986). Later, they seem to have 'forgotten how to listen to people' (Shooter, 2002). Instead of carrying on personal conversations with patients, they conduct interrogations, focussing on symptoms of disease and ignoring what patients say about themselves and their struggle to cope with their illnesses (Weston & Lipkin, 1989). They become more doctor-centred (Haidet *et al.*, 2002), and less empathic (Poole & Sanson-Fisher, 1979). Disiker & Michiellute's study (1981) suggested that the net effect of medical experience, both basic and clinical, is to produce a very small negative change in empathy.

Students learn through personal interaction and observation of clinicians as well as through formal lectures and ward teaching. The theories they learn about how doctors should interact with patients are influenced by the reality of the practice that they see around them. Kurtz *et al.* (2005) state that the way learners themselves are treated has a greater impact than any aspect of the formal curriculum. They also point out that many practitioners and teachers of medical students and residents still use few techniques other than a barrage of close-ended questions. Junior doctors are in practice responsible for much of the communication with hospital inpatients, relatives and carers, even though they are the least experienced and knowledgeable members of the medical team (RCP, 1997).

A survey of 5,330 doctors recently qualified in the UK asked whether their experience at medical school had prepared them well for the jobs they had undertaken so far. Only 4.3% strongly agreed, and 32% agreed that their training had prepared them well for the jobs they had undertaken so far; 22.5% neither agreed nor disagreed; 29.7% disagreed and 11.6% strongly disagreed (Goldacre *et al.*, 2003). Differences between medical schools were large, ranging from 19.8% strongly agreeing or agreeing at one medical school to 73% at another (Goldacre *et al.*, 2003). Wass (2005) reports that 'this variation reflects the fact that UK medical schools are free to develop their own courses and assessments in line with GMC recommendations. There is no common curriculum.' Cohen *et al.* (2005) noted that despite widespread training in medical school, some students and doctors have important deficiencies which, if not addressed, can lead to harm for patients and difficulties with colleagues.

What do patients want to talk to doctors about?

There do seem to be important differences between the topics that a patient wants to talk about to their doctor, and those that the doctor wants the patient to talk about. Each has a separate agenda. Levenstein *et al.* (1989) defined the patient's agenda in terms of ideas, expectations and feelings, and the doctor's agenda in terms of the correct diagnosis of the patient's complaints.

Patients often have more than one concern. However, doctors, in their search for the primary 'presenting complaint,' may assume that patients only have one concern; that the first mentioned concern is the most important and that this has been voiced at the outset. Silverman *et al.* (2005) quote a number of studies from a variety of settings, including primary care, paediatrics and internal medicine, in which the mean number of concerns ranged from 1.2 to 3.9 in both new and return visits (Starfield *et al.* 1981: Good & Good 1982; Wasserman *et al.* 1984; Greenfield *et al.* 1985).

Stewart *et al.* (1979) showed that 54% of patients' complaints and 45% of their concerns were not elicited. Maguire *et al.* (1996a) found that only a minority of health professionals identified more than 60% of their patients' main concerns.

It seems that the patient's full agenda is frequently not discovered. The doctor often redirects the interview after eliciting the first concern, leaving the patient insufficient time or opportunity to fully disclose all concerns. In a study of patients' unvoiced agendas in general practice consultations, Barry *et al.* (2000) found that only four of 35 patients voiced all their agendas in consultation. Most commonly voiced were symptoms and requests for diagnoses and prescriptions. The most common unvoiced items were: worries about possible diagnosis and what the future holds; ideas about what is wrong; side effects; not wanting a prescription; and information relating to social context. Agenda items that were not raised in the consultation often led to specific problem outcomes (for example, major misunderstandings), unwanted prescriptions, non-use of prescriptions, and non-adherence to treatment.

Barsky (1981) showed that patients' 'hidden agendas' may surface in the closing minutes of the visit as 'new problems' if they are not discussed earlier. These new problems are often emotionally charged for the patient, reflecting fear of conditions such as heart disease or cancer. Patients report waiting for the 'right' moment or opportunity to present their 'real' problems.

White *et al.* (1994) found that 21% of patients in primary care introduced new problems, not previously discussed, in the closing moments of the medical visit. They concluded that orienting patients in the flow of the visit, assessing patient beliefs, checking for understanding, and addressing emotions and psychosocial issues early on might decrease the number of new problems in the final moments of the visit.

It seems likely that there are particular topics that patients find it easier to talk to doctors about, such as problems which they have already discussed; physical symptoms that are not frightening, intimate or embarrassing; symptoms which are resolving. More difficult conversations might involve new problems; embarrassing physical symptoms, sexual concerns; psychological issues; side effects of treatment; issues of non-compliance, dissatisfaction or complaint; or where there is disagreement between doctor and patient on diagnosis or management.

Beckman *et al.* (1989) quote Burack & Carpenter (1983) who found that patients typically wait to share psychosocial concerns until late in the visit. Campion *et al.* (1992) showed that the least likely topics for patients to talk about were their social and emotional agendas.

Hargie & Dickson (2004) quote Parrott *et al.* (2000) who state that 'in order for patients to fully disclose, the most important prerequisite is the sensitivity shown by health caregivers which will guide patients in their decision-making about whether to tell the whole truth, or only that part which the caregiver seems most receptive to hearing.' Wissow *et al.* (1994) studied the interview style of paediatricians, and found that specifically asking questions about psychosocial issues, making supportive statements, and listening attentively increased the disclosure of sensitive information.

It is clear that the doctor's use of language and manner of questioning significantly affects the degree to which the patient is able to share their concerns. Beckman *et al.* (1989) quote Bass and Cohen (1982) who found that when patients were asked 'What worries you about this problem?' the majority of patients responded with, 'I'm not worried.' When the same patients were asked, 'What concerns you about the problem?' more than a third voiced previously unrecognised concerns.

In a similar way, the doctor's response influences what beliefs and explanations the patient will be able to introduce into the discussion. Silverman *et al.* (2005) quote Tuckett *et al.* (1985) who found that 26% of patients spontaneously offered an explanation of their symptoms to the doctor. However when patients did express their views only 7% of doctors actively encouraged their patients to elaborate, 13% listened passively and 81% made no effort to listen or deliberately interrupted.

Frankel & Beckman (1989) quote various studies which have shown that patients are more satisfied during the interview when they have an opportunity to share their opinions (Stewart *et al.*, 1984), to ask questions (Roter, 1977), and when doctors show warmth (Francis *et al.*, 1969) and empathy (Wasserman *et al.*, 1984). Despite this, Beckman *et al.* (1989) report West (1983) and Frankel's (1987) observation that patient opportunities to ask questions in primary care were infrequent.

Langewitz *et al.* (1998) noted various studies showing that 50% of patients in outpatient General Internal Medicine do not get what they want from a single consultation (Kravitz *et al.*, 1994; Sanchez-Menegay & Stalder, 1994; Joos *et al.*, 1993). 75% of patients in Tuckett *et al.*'s study (1985) had specific doubts or questions during their medical visits that they did not mention to the doctor; and Roter & Hall (2006) noted that 'it was not unusual for a patient to feel alarmed and confused after leaving the doctor's office because of failures to understand what the doctor was talking about.'

Perhaps not surprisingly, doctors and patients often disagree about the nature of the main complaint. Starfield *et al.* (1981) found that agreement leads to better outcomes and problem resolution, yet in 50% of visits the patient and the doctor did not agree on the nature of the presenting problem. Beckman & Frankel (1984) quote a study by Burack & Carpenter (1983) which found that the patient's chief complaint agreed with the doctor's determination of the patient's primary problem in 76% of somatic but only 6% of psychosocial problems.

What do doctors want patients to talk about?

The doctor's agenda is directed towards finding out enough relevant medical information from the patient in order to make the right diagnosis. The doctor usually makes several assumptions: that the patient has presented with symptoms which have an underlying physical cause; that the doctor must make a diagnosis and formulate a treatment plan; and that the patient will be satisfied with this.

Hampton *et al.* (1975) studied referrals to medical outpatients, and found that in 82% of new patients, the diagnosis that was finally accepted was made after reading the referral letter and taking the history. Peterson *et al.* (1992) found that in 76% of medical outpatients, the history led to the final diagnosis. Maguire (2000) stated that the history contributes far more to accurate diagnosis than do medical investigations, and that the medical interview is crucial for identifying the exact problems for which patients need help.

The doctor's aim, then, is to gather information. However, Langewitz *et al.* (1998) found that only 55 to 69% of medical information was identified by internal medicine residents during medical consultations. Roter & Hall (1987) investigated experienced primary care practitioners during simulated patient encounters. They found that physicians elicited only slightly more than 50% of the medical information considered important according to expert consensus, with a range from 9% to 85%.

A doctor thinks within the biomedical model and would like the patient to do the same. Ideally, s/he would like the patient to speak factually, objectively and succinctly, in order to make a diagnosis as quickly and efficiently as possible. Doctors fear that patients, left to their own devices, will talk for far too long. However, it has in fact been shown that doctors always talk more than patients. Roter & Hall (2006) found that during medical visits the average amount of physician contribution to the medical dialogue is 60%, whereas patients contribute 40%. Information that does not directly lead to diagnosis may be seen as irrelevant, such as the patient's feelings, their beliefs about symptoms, and the impact of their illness on his life.

Tate (2007) states that doctors rarely talk to patients about the consequences of their illnesses. He quotes a study of oncologists in 1996 which found that 'the doctors used closed questions and seldom gave the patients space to initiate any discussion. Only 1% of their talk was related to their concerns. Emotional well-being was rarely probed. There were almost no social questions from the doctors, and the researchers found that the level of expressed empathy from the doctors was as low as 1%.'

Rogers & Todd (2000) taped 74 consultations between cancer patients and doctors and found that doctor-initiated questions were prominent. Over three-quarters were closed questions which focused narrowly on limited physical aspects of the patient's pain. They found that doctors tightly controlled the agenda to focus on pain which was amenable to radiotherapy, chemotherapy, surgery, or hormone manipulation. Various communication tactics were used to avoid talk of other problems. Interestingly, Shilling *et al.* (2003) found that clinicians were less satisfied following consultations with patients being treated palliatively.

If the patient becomes upset, this can be time-consuming and may provoke uncomfortable feelings even for the doctor. Patients may express emotions that the doctor finds difficult to deal with, such as fear, anger, or hopelessness.

Levinson *et al.* (2000) conducted a qualitative study of 116 visits to 54 primary care physicians and 62 surgeons. They postulated that patients often present clues (direct or indirect comments about personal aspects of their lives or their emotions) during conversations with their physicians. They found that physicians responded positively to patient emotions in 38% of cases in surgery and 21% in primary care, but more frequently they missed opportunities to adequately acknowledge patients' feelings. Visits with missed opportunities tended to be longer than visits with a positive response.

Batenburg *et al.* (1999) conducted a study in Holland and found that final-year students preferring general practice as a specialty as well as vocational trainees in general practice showed more patient-centred attitudes than surgery trainees and students preferring surgery.

Silverman *et al.* (2005) report that:

> *Stewart (1985) looked at 133 interviews in primary care and compared their patient-centeredness score with the length of consultation. Low scores average 7.8 minutes, intermediate scores 10.9 minutes, high scores 8.5 minutes. Stewart concluded that doctors can expect to take longer while they learn the skills, however, doctors who had mastered the patient-centred approach took little extra time compared with doctors who did not employ these techniques.*

Langewitz *et al.* (1998) reported that 'physicians have difficulties listening to patients; they underestimate their information needs (Sardell & Trierweiler, 1993) and their functional disabilities (Calkins *et al.*, 1991).' Turner and Kelly (2000) observed that the emotional dimensions of chronic conditions are often overlooked. Their view is that doctors 'may be well-equipped for the biomedical aspects of care, but not for the challenges of understanding the psychological, social and cultural dimensions of illness and health.'

The ability to listen to patients and the willingness to make attempts to understand how they feel are both aspects of empathy. Studies have reported that doctors dominate interviews (Squier, 1990); they show low levels of empathy (Reynolds & Scott, 2000), and become defensive (Sloane, 1993). They use language that is incomprehensible to patients (Svarstad, 1974 in Roter & Hall, 2006), and consistently overestimate patients' understanding (Tate, 2007). The language doctors use is often unclear, both as regards the use of jargon and in relation to a lack of the expected shared meanings of relatively common terms (Simpson *et al.*, 1991).

How much do patients want to be involved in decision-making?

It is clear that in order to make an informed decision about treatment, a patient needs to be given a clear explanation of the options available. This information must be provided in a form that is understandable to the patient. Discussion needs to take place, both about the particular diagnosis of that individual's case, and about the wider issues in relation to treatments available; risks, benefits, and side effects. The doctor needs to check that the patient has understood the information, agrees with the diagnosis, and has been given an opportunity to ask questions. A patient is much more likely to adhere to a management plan that has been discussed and agreed.

Levinson *et al.* (2005) undertook a population-based study which showed that people vary substantially in how involved they wish to be in decisions about their care. They found that those over 45 years of age, and those in poorer health, tended to prefer a physician-directed style of decision-making.

Arora & McHorney (2000) found that 69% of patients preferred to leave the medical decision to their doctors. Younger people, and those with better education, preferred an active role. Women were more likely to be active than men, both in participating in treatment decisions and asking questions. McKinstry (2000) found in general practice that patients' desire to take part in decision-making varied, depending on the presenting problem but also the age, social class, and educational level of the patient.

Brody *et al.* (1989) found that 47% of general medical patients reported playing an active role and 53% a passive role. Active patients reported less discomfort, greater alleviation of symptoms, and more improvement in their general medical condition one week after the visits than did passive patients. Active patients also reported less concern, a greater sense of control of their illnesses, and more satisfaction with their physicians one day after the visit.

Charles *et al.* (2000) make the distinction between a paternalistic and an informed approach. In an informed, or shared, approach, the doctor provides information about treatment options, benefits and risks, and, together with the patient, develops a treatment plan which is consistent with the patient's values and preferences.

Faden *et al.* (1981) studied doctors who treated seizures and patients (or parents of patients) with this disorder. They found that patients preferred far more detailed disclosures than doctors routinely offer, and wanted extensive information regarding risks and alternative therapy. Doctors were likely to disclose only risks with a relatively high probability of occurrence and provided little information about alternative therapies. Patients and parents were also much more likely than physicians to believe that the final decision concerning therapy should rest with the patient.

Waitzkin (1984) stated that patients frequently complain about the information they do and do not receive. In other words, patients may be receiving either information that they do not want, or not being given the opportunity to find out the information that they do want. Waitzkin's finding was that patients almost always want as much information as possible and doctors frequently do not realise this.

Waitzkin (1985) analysed a sample of 336 encounters from several outpatient settings in the US and revealed that doctors spent little time informing their patients, overestimated the time they did spend and underestimated patients' desire for information: in only 6% of cases did they overestimate it. In encounters that averaged 16.5 minutes, the mean time spent by doctors in information giving was 1.3 minutes, or about 9% of the total interaction time. Patients spent a small amount of time questioning, on average, 8 seconds, or about 1% of the total time available. Doctors estimated that they devoted 8.9 minutes to information giving, rather than the observed time of 1.3 minutes.

Silverman *et al.* (2005) quote Kindelan & Kent (1987), who 'in a UK study in general practice, found that patients most wanted information about the diagnosis, prognosis and causation of their condition. Doctors greatly underestimated their patients' desire for this information, and overestimated their desire for information about treatment and drug therapy.'

Many doctors follow a set routine in delivering information, without tailoring this to the individual patient's information needs. Patients' needs for information may change through the course of an illness. Often the consequences and likely prognosis without treatment is not adequately discussed, or not discussed at all. One reason suggested for this is that health professionals may themselves lack knowledge of treatment options and their effects (Coulter *et al.*, 1999); thus they may not be good at communicating about risk. Smith (2003) states that 'when doctors made decisions for patients – as many still do – they didn't need to communicate risk. Now, it is increasingly one of their central tasks.'

Patient focus groups organised by Coulter *et al.* (1999) reported considerable dissatisfaction with their experiences of communication with health professionals. Most patients wanted much more information about their condition than they had been given. Many did not feel that they had been offered any choices about their treatment and some had not realised that there were other options. The researchers concluded that patients cannot express informed preferences unless they are given sufficient and appropriate information, including detailed explanations about their condition and the likely outcomes with and without treatment.

Leydon *et al.* (2000) found that all oncology patients in a study in London wanted basic information on diagnosis and treatment, but not all wanted further information at all stages of their illness. The Royal College of Physicians (1997) reported that studies of cancer patients have repeatedly revealed large gaps in their understanding of the nature of their illness, their prognosis and their treatment.

In studies of general practice, Savage & Armstrong (1990) found that patients whom the doctor judged to have a chronic illness, patients who judged themselves to have a psychological illness, and those who only wanted advice did not prefer a directing style. McKinstry (2000) found that when patients believed they may have had more insight into the problem than their doctor, such as for depression or lifestyle, more preferred to help decide their management. McKinstry (2000) points out, however, that doctors need to determine for individual patients how much involvement in decision-making they want.

What is good communication?

Growing evidence suggests that doctors who focus on the patient as well as the disease obtain more accurate historical data, increase patient adherence, and build more effective patient-physician relationships (Platt *et al.*, 2001). Good communication helps the patient to recall information and comply with treatment instructions, and leads to improved patient satisfaction (Hulsman, 2002; Maguire & Pitceathly, 2002).

Good communication may improve patient health and outcomes. Better communication and dialogue has a beneficial effect in promoting better emotional health, resolution of symptoms and pain control (Meryn, 1998).

In recent times, various systems have evolved which provide a framework for good communication. For example, Griffin *et al.* (2004) aim at:

- Increasing the patient's contribution at all stages of the clinical interview
- Increasing the practitioner's ability to elicit and integrate the patient's views with the biomedical view.

Many of the recommendations made by the Bristol Inquiry urged doctors to include patients as active participants in their own care, and to:

- Involve patients (or their parents) in decisions.
- Keep patients (or parents) informed.
- Provide patients with counselling and support.
- Gain informed consent for all procedures and processes.
- Elicit feedback from patients and listen to their views.
- Be open and candid when adverse events occur (Coulter, 2002a).

DiMatteo & Chow (1995) suggest the following steps for enhancing compliance and improving communication:

1. Explain to patients their diagnosis and possible causes.

2. Listen to the patient's fears and frustrations. Encourage patients to ask questions and to describe personal expectations for treatment, including effects on lifestyle.

3. Answer patient's questions. Address unrealistic expectations.

4. Suggest a treatment approach that may fit the patient's expressed preferences. Describe expected benefits and costs, risks, and expected outcomes, and other possible courses of action, including no treatment.

5. Obtain patient feedback concerning benefits of treatment along with understanding and acceptance of risk. Devise methods to address concerns.

6. Discuss with the patient in detail when and how medication will be taken. Correct misunderstandings.

7. Work with the patient to elicit commitment to following the treatment regimen. If the patient appears hesitant, return to step 2. Simplifying and reminding will not help a patient follow a regimen that he or she does not believe in.

8. Work with the patient to build supports for and reduce barriers to the regimen.

9. Revisit the issue of when and how the regimen will implemented, and attempt to anticipate problems and suggest solutions.

What is poor communication?

Sometimes communication between doctors and patients simply fails. A Consumers' Association survey of patients' first visits to a consultant showed that 30% felt inhibited from asking questions, often because they expected to be told automatically. Others felt a need to 'protect' the specialist who seemed rushed or under pressure (RCP, 1997).

Ley (1988) points out that patients often do not understand or remember what they are told. What clinicians say is often not in understandable or memorable form. Furthermore, because patients do not provide feedback in the form of questions, clinicians remain unaware of their faults in communicating.

There is evidence that 'many physicians listen poorly, miss vital non-verbal cues, misdiagnose emotional and mental conditions, and respond with a lack of understanding and insight' (Bub, 2006).

Byrne & Long (1976) examined consultations which had gone wrong, and found that doctors overuse reassurance, including when they have assumed they understand the problem exactly, and then use reassurance to justify their own assumptions.

Heath (1984) showed that when doctors attempt to read the patient's records and listen to the patient at the same time, they frequently miss or forget what the patient tells them. If the doctor reads the notes while patients are talking, patients stop until eye contact is resumed, or try to regain the doctor's attention through body movement.

It may be that a patient is very anxious, in which case the anxiety needs to be addressed and their concerns explored. Some doctors do not feel comfortable doing this; they may also tend to avoid asking about issues which they think will trigger strong emotion. Byrne & Long (1976) found that 'any intrusion of feeling or risk of emotive content was rapidly countered by a closed question about some new issue.' Maguire (2000) stated that 'doctors keep interviews emotionally neutral by ignoring cues about patients' worries and emotions, which can lead patients to avoid mentioning key problems.'

The Royal College of Physicians (1997) reports a variety of reasons for poor communication, including the inability of doctors to recognise patients' concerns; the tendency to overlook the need of patients to be heard and to be given clear explanations, and the failure to take psychological and social factors into account. They acknowledge the contribution of lack of time, pressure of work, constant interruptions, stress or over-tiredness. However, attention is also drawn to specific inappropriate and authoritarian attitudes that may give rise to poor communication: a fear of patients knowing too much; a belief that patients 'need not worry themselves' or cannot understand; hostility and impatience towards assertive patients; a desire to retain control.

Byrne & Long in 1976 reported that about 3% of the consultations which they studied in general practice contained elements of negative behaviour by doctors, especially in response to patient initiatives which were not appreciated by the doctor. Examples were:

- Rejecting patient offers: 'Let's concentrate on your rash, shall we?'
- Reinforcing self-position: 'I am the doctor…'
- Denying the patient: 'I do not wish to have you on my list'.
- Refusing patient ideas: 'No, I don't think that will help at all'.
- Evading patient questions: 'Let's not worry about that…'
- Not listening: some doctors admit that some patients are so irritating that the best defence is not to listen.
- Refusing to respond to feeling.
- Confused noise: in consultations which are not working well, the doctor and patient are talking at the same time and neither stops to listen to what the other is saying.

There are many possible reasons why a consultation does not run smoothly. Doctors may worry about their own competence, and fear inadequacy or admitting their own ignorance, therefore avoiding seeking advice from more competent colleagues (RCP, 1997). Experienced clinicians may have developed ingrained patterns of behaviour. Lack of insight may prevent doctors from remedying their weaknesses, even when they are accurately identified (Kinnersley & Edwards, 2008).

Outcome studies

Patient satisfaction
Korsch (1989) defines satisfaction, for both patient and doctor, as 'a short-term outcome of the medical interaction which can be measured immediately following an encounter.' On the other hand, 'intermediate outcomes such as compliance, anxiety reduction, or increased self-esteem and confidence may take time to become evident. Finally, symptom resolution and changes in functional status and quality of life, as well as decreases in morbidity and mortality, are long-term outcomes that may need a relatively longer period of follow-up and monitoring.'

In terms of short-term outcome, various studies have investigated the level of patient satisfaction following a consultation. A Consumers' Association survey of 262 people who had made a first visit to see a hospital consultant revealed that about 85% were satisfied with what they had been told by the specialist, and of those about 50% were very satisfied (RCP, 1997). Jackson *et al.* (2001) conducted a study in a general medicine walk in clinic, and found that 53% of patients were fully satisfied with their care. Shilling *et al.* (2003) reported that satisfaction for cancer patients was related to patients' age, psychological morbidity and most significantly, satisfaction with the length of wait in clinic.

Patient satisfaction is also related to the amount of information that patients are given. Specifically, general practice patients wanted explanations of the likely cause, diagnosis and prognosis of their condition (Kindelan & Kent, 1987, in Silverman *et al.*, 2005). In Jackson *et al.*'s (2001) study in the medical walk-in clinic, '98% of patients had at least one pre-visit expectation, including a desire for a causal explanation (80%), anticipated time for recovery (62%), medication prescription (66%), diagnostic test (56%), or subspecialty referral (47%).' In general, patients are more satisfied if these expectations are met, or if the doctor at least asks about their expectations (Eisenthal & Lazare, 1976; Eisenthal *et al.*, 1979).

One of the problems, according to Meryn (1998), is that 'doctors and patients have different views on what makes good and effective communication. Patients want more and better information about their problem and the outcome, more openness about the side effects of treatment, relief of pain and emotional distress, and advice on what they can do for themselves.'

Providing information is important not only in terms of improving satisfaction. It has also been shown to be associated with improved resolution of symptoms, reduced emotional distress, improved physiological status, reduced use of analgesia, reduced length of hospital stay, and improved quality of life (Kaplan *et al.*, 1989; Fallowfield *et al.*, 1994; Roter *et al.*, 1995; Stewart, 1995; Kinnersley *et al.*, 2008).

However, Maguire *et al.* (1989) found that few doctors explained the purpose of the interview or the time available, and in only 25% of visits did the doctors negotiate about treatment.

It appears that patients are frequently dissatisfied with the quality and amount of information they receive (Ley, 1988). Patients complain more about communication with doctors than about any other aspect of their care (Richards, 1990), the commonest complaint being that doctors do not listen to them (Meryn, 1998). There is evidence that 'more questioning on biomedical topics is associated with lower satisfaction (Bertakis *et al.*, 1991; Roter *et al.*, 1987), whereas psychosocial questioning is very well received by patients' (Roter & Hall, 2006). A survey of 5,150 patients recently discharged from hospital revealed that 34% of them had not been told the results of tests (Tate, 2007).

Other issues are also important to satisfaction. Hall *et al.* (1988) in a meta-analysis of 412 independent studies reported that patient satisfaction was related most dramatically to the amount of information given by doctors. It was also related to greater technical and interpersonal competence, more partnership building, more immediate and positive nonverbal behaviour, more social conversation, more positive talk, less negative talk and more communication overall. Asking questions showed no relation to satisfaction. Coulter (2002b) quotes a systematic review of general practice published in 1998 by Wensing *et al.*, in which patients rated humaneness most highly, followed by competence/accuracy, involvement in decisions, and time for care.

Roberts *et al.* (1994) conducted a study six months after the interview in which women were diagnosed with breast cancer. They found that psychological adjustment was predicted by physician behaviour during the cancer diagnostic interview. The physician's caring attitude was perceived by the women as most important, with information-giving a much weaker component. Specific surgeons' behaviours which facilitate patient adjustment include expressing empathy, allowing sufficient time for patients to absorb the cancer diagnosis, providing information, and engaging the patient in treatment decision-making.

Mager & Andrykowski (2002) conducted a study to explore relationships between breast cancer survivors' experiences during the diagnostic consultation and their subsequent long-term psychological adjustment. They found that women's perceptions of physicians' interpersonal skills during the diagnostic consultation were associated with later psychological adjustment.

Jackson *et al.* (2001) quote studies which have shown that 'patients rate health outcomes of care as the most important determinant of satisfaction (Jatulis *et al.*, 1997), and that patients with greater functional impairment are less likely to be satisfied with the care they receive (Cleary & McNeil, 1988; Williams & Calnan, 1991).' However, various researchers express reservations about the reliability of satisfaction data because it is known that patients are reluctant to be critical (Jackson *et al.*, 2001; Shilling *et al.*, 2003) and are sometimes fearful of provoking a worsening of their care (Shilling *et al.*, 2003).

Patient compliance/concordance

There has recently been a shift in attitudes towards decision-making in prescribing, moving away from the old concept of compliance, which was thought to be authoritarian and disempowering for patients, towards the new concept of concordance, which incorporates new values such as shared decision-making, partnership, and respect for patient autonomy. Compliance refers to the following of instructions, whereas concordance is an agreement about whether and how medicines are to be taken (Marinker & Shaw, 2003).

The term concordance, introduced in 1997 by the Royal Pharmaceutical Society, was incorporated into the *Expert Patient* (DH, 2001b) and endorsed by the Department of Health in 2002. The Medicines Partnership Task Force was set up to implement concordance in the NHS. The principles were that 'doctors should provide clear and sufficiently detailed information to patients in order that the wishes of the patient can be incorporated into the process of prescribing' (Heath, 2003).

According to the *Expert Patient* (DH, 2001b), concordance is an agreement reached after negotiation between a patient and a healthcare professional. Doctor and patient discuss why treatment is needed and what options are available. The doctor explores the patient's preferences, and finds out what the patient has learned about the consequences of taking or not taking prescribed medications. Many patients have experience of which drugs suit them best, or which have least side-effects. They have found through trial and error what happens if they do or don't take a particular medication or combination of drugs. On the basis of these discussions, patient and doctor decide together whether a drug will be used or not.

Recent studies have shown that this is at yet an ideal to be aimed for. Cockburn & Pit (1997) found that doctors often fail to understand patients' preferences. Elwyn *et al.* (2003) state that 'doctors often do not name the drug they prescribe, or describe how new drugs differ from those previously prescribed; they do not usually check patients' understanding, explore their concerns, or discuss patients' ability to follow a treatment plan.' Coulter (2002b) reports that 'there is little evidence that general practitioners and patients share decision making.'

Cockburn & Pit (1997), in a study of general practice in Australia, found that medicines were prescribed in 50% of cases, most likely to patients with respiratory, skin, digestive, or psychological conditions. The strongest predictor of medication prescription was not the patient's actual expectation but the doctors' opinions about their expectations. Of the people whom the general practitioner considered to expect medication, 80% received a prescription.

The guidelines on medicines adherence (NICE, 2009) state that failure to adhere to a treatment regime usually results from a breakdown in the initial negotiation process. If the patient is not fully convinced that the medication is necessary and that the benefits will outweigh the risks, then it is quite likely that s/he will not take it as directed.

The doctor may simply assume at the next visit that the patient has followed the prescribed regimen, and may neglect to ask questions such as; 'Have you been taking the medication? How often do you take it? Are there times when you forget it?' Once the doctor has established that the patient is not taking the medication all the time, s/he can then explore with the patient what might improve their concordance: 'What influences whether you take it or not? Is there anything else you need to know in order to decide whether this medication is the best treatment for you?'

If the doctor is unaware that the patient has not taken the drugs as prescribed, either in terms of dosage or frequency, then there are any number of inaccurate conclusions to reach; that the drug has not worked; that the illness is worsening; that the patient needs a higher dose of the same drug; that the patient needs a different or additional drug; that s/he is dealing with a treatment-resistant case.

Marinker & Shaw (2003) make the interesting point that 'doctors seem to behave as though non-compliance is a problem for other doctors. When the medicines that doctors prescribe fail to produce the benefit they expect, they often respond by varying the dose or selecting an alternative medicine' – rather than asking whether the patient has in fact taken them!

Around one-third of people in the United Kingdom receive long-term medication (Dowell *et al.*, 2002). However, it is well known that many patients do not take the medicines prescribed. The figure of 50% suggested by Haynes *et al.* (1996) is often quoted as a typical rate of adherence. A recent meta-analysis (DiMatteo, 2004a) of treatment prescribed by non-psychiatric doctors showed an average non-adherence rate of 24.8%. Adherence was found to be highest in HIV disease, arthritis, gastrointestinal disorders, and cancer and lowest in pulmonary disease and diabetes.

A review of the literature reveals that the amount of information that patients receive directly affects their ability to make treatment decisions. The Royal College of Physicians (1997) states that inadequate explanation is the most frequent cause of poor compliance, as patients may be unwilling or unable to comply with suggested treatments if they do not understand the reasons for what has been proposed. Kurtz *et al.* (2005) report that 'doctors overestimate how much they discuss the risks of medication (Makoul *et al.*, 1995); Svarstad (1974) found no discussion at all in 20 % of cases, and no information about the name or purpose of the drug in 30%.'

Ley (1988) suggested that adherence was determined by such factors as understanding, recall and satisfaction. Kessels (2003) states that 40–80% of medical information provided by healthcare practitioners is forgotten immediately, particularly if the patient is old or anxious. Kessels (2003) quotes that women at risk for breast cancer remembered less information if the physician made a worried impression (thus increasing the level of distress) (Shapiro *et al.*, 1992), whilst for rheumatology patients, almost half of the information they recalled was incorrect (Anderson *et al.*, 1979).

O'Connor *et al.* (1999) found that when patients were provided with unbiased, evidence based information about treatment options, likely outcomes and self care, they usually made rational choices that were often more conservative and involved less risk than their doctors would choose.

Ferner (2003) quotes that a meta-analysis of treatment of hypertension showed that '95% of patients who take their tablets for five years will be no better off (Mulrow *et al.*, 2000); also that two thirds of older patients prescribed a statin for coronary artery disease give up treatment within two years (Jackevicius *et al.*, 2002).' Newell *et al.* (1998) quote Shapiro (1987) who estimated that up to one-third of patients will abandon chemotherapy prematurely as a result of physical side-effects and psychosocial symptoms such as disrupted work, relationships, social and sexual activities, and financial pressures, despite the potentially life-threatening consequences of such action.

Primary among explanations for poor adherence are poor provider-patient relationships in which patients misunderstand the treatment regimen and in which trust and caring are not communicated by the provider (Waitzkin, 1984). Providers who have a controlling, paternalistic manner give patients little opportunity to make a personal commitment to the regimen (DiMatteo & Chow, 1995). Jones (2003) reports that although 'doctors say that not taking drugs means poorer health outcomes, patients argue that only they can know what works for them and what doesn't'. Travaline *et al.* (2005) point out that effective patient-physician communication can improve a patient's health as quantifiably as many drugs.

Improving adherence is just as much a challenge for patients as it is for health professionals (Van Dulmen *et al.*, 2008). As the National Institute for Health and Clinical Excellence guidance (2009) states, the patient has the right to decide not to take a medicine, even if the doctor does not agree with the decision, as long as the patient has the capacity to make an informed decision and has been provided with the necessary information. Some patients may make the perfectly legitimate choice not to take medication. Other patients may not take medication due to involuntary factors such as physical or mental incapacity, social isolation, or the difficulty of maintaining the regimen on a daily basis (Marinker & Shaw, 2003). Patients at greatest risk for non-adherence to treatment include: those who are most severely ill with serious diseases (DiMatteo *et al.*, 2007); those from families in conflict (DiMatteo, 2004b); and those who are depressed (DiMatteo *et al.*, 2000).

Dowell *et al.* (2002) identified four problematic issues for patients using treatment suboptimally: understanding, acceptance, level of personal control, and motivation. Identifying and discussing these barriers improved management for some. Haynes *et al.* (1996) summarised the results of randomised controlled trials of interventions to help patients follow prescriptions, and found that even the most effective did not lead to substantial improvements in adherence. Keeping patients in care was the most important adherence intervention.

Health outcomes

Levinson *et al.* (2005) quote various studies which show that patients who are knowledgeable about their condition (Kaplan *et al.*, 1989; Greenfield *et al.*, 1985: Greenfield *et al.*, 1988), or are involved in decision-making (Deber *et al.*, 1996) enjoy improved health outcomes. 'A study by Tuckett (1976) found that when patients have been informed by their doctor as to what to expect they recover more quickly than when they are simply passive recipients of treatment' (RCP, 1997).

Effective communication skills have been correlated to positive outcomes such as adherence to therapy, understanding of treatment risks (Travaline *et al.*, 2005); biological outcomes in chronic disease, and patient satisfaction (Levinson & Lurie, 2004). Patients who ask questions, elicit treatment options, express opinions, and state preferences about treatment have measurably better health outcomes than patients who do not (Kaplan *et al.*, 1989). Patients who feel that they have participated in decision-making are more likely to follow through on those decisions than those who do not (Kaplan *et al.*, 1996).

There are several frequently quoted studies on health outcomes related to communication skills. The Headache Study Group (1986) found that the best outcomes after one year of follow-up were in patients who felt they had been given sufficient opportunity to tell the doctor all they wanted to say about their headaches on the initial visit (Weston & Brown, 1989).

Stewart (1995) reviewed randomised controlled trials and found that:

> *In 16 of 21 studies the quality of communication both in the history-taking and discussion of the management plan influenced patient health outcomes. The outcomes affected were, in descending order of frequency, emotional health, symptom resolution, function, physiologic measures (ie blood pressure and blood sugar level) and pain control. Most of the studies demonstrated a correlation between effective physician-patient communication and improved patient health outcomes.*

Coulter *et al.* (1999) quote various studies investigating the benefits of shared decision-making:

- Patients with hypertension benefit if they are allowed to adopt an active rather than a passive role in treatment (England & Evans, 1992).
- Patients with breast cancer suffer less depression and anxiety if they are treated by doctors who adopt a participative consultation style (Fallowfield *et al.*, 1990).
- Patients who are more actively involved in discussion about the management of their diabetes achieve better blood sugar control (Kaplan *et al.*, 1989).

Kaplan *et al.* (1996) quote various studies of patients with hypertension (Kaplan *et al.*, 1989), non-insulin-dependent diabetes mellitus, peptic ulcer disease, and rheumatoid arthritis, which showed that patients whose physicians were less controlling (or more participatory) had better functional status and lower follow-up glycosylated haemoglobin levels, blood pressure, and arthritis severity than patients of less participatory physicians.

Shilling *et al.* (2003) report various studies on cancer diagnosis which showed that women who were not satisfied with the information given at time of diagnosis adjusted less well to their cancer and its treatment (Fallowfield, 1990), and that patients who rated their doctors' discussion of treatment options highly had better psychological adjustment to a cancer diagnosis (Butow *et al.*, 1996).

In a review of evidence on patient- doctor communication, Stewart *et al.* (1999) found that the following aspects of communication about the management plan significantly influenced health outcomes:

- Patient being encouraged to ask questions.
- Provision of clear information.
- Willingness of doctor to share decision-making.
- Agreement between patient and doctor about the problem and the plan.

Lang *et al.* (2002) report that the patient's perspective on illness (PPI) surfaces spontaneously in only about one fourth of medical interviews, despite the fact that numerous authors have noted that facilitating patients' sharing of their perspective results in improved disease outcomes and higher levels of patient satisfaction and adherence with therapy (Kaplan *et al.*, 1989; Starfield *et al.*, 1981).

'Physician solicitation of patient perspectives has a positive impact on patient trust, and also satisfies a basic human need for expression that may have therapeutic value' (Haidet & Paterniti, 2003). Hargie & Dickson (2004) state that 'in a comprehensive review of the research on a range of illnesses (such as cardiovascular diseases, HIV, cancer, etc.) Tardy (2000) found considerable evidence to show that self-disclosure has positive effects on health. One reason for this is that disclosure has been shown to boost immunological functioning (Petrie *et al.* 1995).' Furthermore, being treated with dignity and being involved in decisions are independently associated with positive outcomes (Beach *et al.*, 2005).

Medical failure

Medicine can fail patients in a number of different ways. Meryn (1998) quotes Richards (1990) who states that 'most complaints by patients and the public about doctors deal with problems of communication not with clinical competency.' Coulter (2002a) states that, in addition, 'failure to take account of the patient's perspective is at the heart of most formal complaints and legal actions. She quotes the survey conducted by Vincent *et al.* (1994)

which found that 'the overwhelming majority of litigants who sued healthcare providers were dissatisfied with the nature and clarity of the explanations they were given and the lack of sympathy displayed by staff after the incident.'

Frenkel & Liebman (2004), former litigators and now mediators and clinical law teachers, state that 'ineffective communication is the single largest factor in producing patient litigation, and good communication, including effective apologies, can avert or help end conflict, especially litigation. Apologies have a potential for healing that is matched only by the difficulty most people have in offering them.'

Levinson *et al.* (1997) state that physician communication styles appear to be associated with the risk of malpractice litigation in the US. They studied primary care physicians, general surgeons, and orthopaedic surgeons, who they classified into no-claims or claims groups based on insurance company records:

> *Significant differences in communication behaviours of no-claims and claims physicians were identified in primary care physicians but not in surgeons. Compared with claims primary care physicians, no-claims primary care physicians used more statements of orientation (educating patients about what to expect and the flow of a visit), laughed and used humour more, tended to use more facilitation (soliciting patients' opinions, checking understanding, and encouraging patients to talk), and spent longer in routine visits.*

Hickson *et al.* (2002) carried out a retrospective cohort study of 645 general and specialist physicians in a large US medical group. They found that 'both patient complaints and risk management events were higher for surgeons than non-surgeons, confirming the results of Sloan *et al.* (1989) who found that 2–8% of internists, obstetricians and surgeons accounted for 75–85% of award and settlement costs.' However, Hickson *et al.* (2002) also showed that a small number of physicians experience a disproportionate share of complaints, malpractice claims and expenses.

Interestingly, unsolicited patient complaints were positively associated with physicians' risk management experiences, ranging from file openings to multiple lawsuits. They concluded that 'risk seems not to be predicted by patient characteristics, illness complexity, or even physicians' technical skills. Instead, risk appears related to patients' dissatisfaction with their physicians' ability to establish rapport, provide access, administer care and treatment consistent with expectations, and communicate effectively.'

Irwin & Richardson (2006) quote Beckman *et al.* (2004) who conducted a study of malpractice cases against a metropolitan medical centre. They found that:

> *The decision to litigate was often associated with a perceived lack of caring and/or collaboration in the delivery of healthcare. Problematic relationship issues between the doctor and patient were identified in 71% of the depositions. These could be categorized by four themes: deserting the patient (32%), devaluing patient and/or family views (29%), delivering information poorly (26%), and failing to understand the patient and/or family perspective (13%). If more attention had been focused on the physician/patient interaction, particularly at the post-outcome consultation, litigation could have been avoided in many of these cases.*

Forster *et al.* (2002) states that:

> *the fear of liability leads to the consequent practice of 'defensive medicine' to avoid lawsuits. In the United States, before 1960 only 1 in 7 physicians were sued throughout their entire career. Today, it is estimated that 1 in 7 are sued every year. In one study by the AMA (1985), 42% of physicians reported that they acted differently in their dealing with patients because of liability concerns; they spent more time with patients, ordered extra tests or procedures, and documented their patient encounters in more detail. We suggest that if physicians improve their communication skills, document the basis for decisions clearly, practice skilled medicine, engage in honest and open discourse with patients, and treat patients and their families respectfully, they can reduce their legal risk. Studies suggest that these aspects of physician performance are the factors that distinguish injured patients who sue from those who do not.*

In the UK, litigation is much less frequent than in the United States. However, similar issues seem to be relevant; risk of complaint and litigation is reduced by patient-centred care: explaining clearly, allowing patients informed choice, involving patients in negotiation and shared decision-making. Clearly communication is at the heart of successful medicine.

Cockburn & Pit (1997) state that 'if doctors are ignorant of patients' values and preferences, patients may receive treatment that is inappropriate to their needs.'

Ley (1998) reports that Oliver *et al.* (1995) found in a study of patients' recall of written consent and information forms that '75% could not name any of their drugs, 26% could not recall the goals of their treatment, and only 15% remembered the 4 side effects they were likely to experience.'

Coulter (2002a) states that 'procedures used to gain informed consent often fall short of the ideal. Many involve a hasty discussion between a patient and a junior doctor, whose sole aim is to get a signature on a form. Options and alternatives are rarely discussed with the patient (or parent), and the "consent" implied by the signature cannot be said to be truly informed (Lavelle-Jones *et al.*, 1993).'

Furthermore, 'patients are often given a biased and highly optimistic picture of the benefits of medical care. Doctors who fail to provide full and balanced information about the risks and uncertainties of procedures and treatments can create unrealistic expectations; these may be the reason for the UK's rising rates of litigation' (Coulter *et al.*, 1999).

As Hurwitz & Vass (2002) write:

> *In the United Kingdom, a series of inquiries has ushered in probably the most sustained investigation and collective appraisal of medical and healthcare institutions since the NHS began. The performance of individual clinicians, laboratory and clinical units, the frequency of medical mistakes, the unacceptability of organ retention practices, and the adequacy of death certification procedures are only a few of many medical activities now subject to intense scrutiny.*

Chapter 3
Communication theory

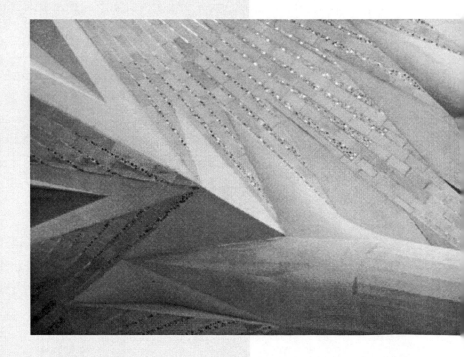

Communication theory

The mechanics of communication

Communication theory is the branch of knowledge that deals with language and other means of conveying or exchanging information. Communication is defined by the New Shorter Oxford English Dictionary as a way of making connections, a means of access between people. In addition to transmission or exchange of information, it also involves succeeding in evoking understanding.

Language, says Groopman (2008), is still the bedrock of clinical practice. Communication is not simply a uni-directional flow, the delivery of a message or a set of instructions. It is a bilateral interaction in which physician and patient discuss the options and weigh the choices (Levinson *et al.*, 2005). It is a means of establishing and developing relationships – with patients and also with colleagues and other members of the healthcare team.

Linguistic skills are not only important for communication and teamwork, but also for decision-making and critical thinking (Holman, 2000). Indeed, the physicians' core clinical skills are interpersonal (Novack *et al.*, 1993). Hargie & Dickson (2004) quote Brooks & Heath (1993) who defined interpersonal communication as 'the process by which information, meanings and feelings are shared by persons through the exchange of verbal and nonverbal messages.'

Communication acts at different levels simultaneously; Watzlawick *et al.* (1967) suggested two separate but interrelated levels of content and relationship. Powers (1995) added in context and the individual or group, to make four tiers of communication (in Littlejohn & Foss, 2005). Content, or subject matter, relates to the topic under discussion. The relationship between the people interacting includes, amongst other things, how each projects their own identity and looks for confirmation of this from the other (Hargie & Dickson, 2004).

From these definitions, it is clear that communication covers a number of different areas, including information giving and receiving; education; understanding; connection and relationship; expression of thoughts and feelings; and enacting a self and group identity. Each of these aspects will be explored later in greater depth.

Models of communication

In order to understand more about how communication works within the health care setting, it is helpful to consider what is known about communication in a wider context. In their book *Theories of Human Communication*, Professors Littlejohn and Foss (2005) present a framework for understanding communication. They quote Craig's (1999) meta-model which divides communication theory into seven traditions: semiotic; phenomenological; cybernetic; sociopsychological; sociocultural; critical; and rhetorical. Their explanations of each of these are of relevance, and have therefore been presented in detail below.

The semiotic tradition

Littlejohn & Foss (2005) explain semiotics as the study of signs and symbols. A branch of this is semantics – what signs stand for. Words are verbal signs and gestures are a form of nonverbal signs. 'Nonverbal signs are paired with language to express subtle, complex meanings. People can communicate if they share meanings, that is, if they have a common understanding of words, grammar, society and culture – if not, then gaps and misunderstandings arise.'

Keller & Carroll (1994) state that doctors learn a diagnostic way of thinking and problem solving, and, during their medical training, it has been estimated that they learn 13,000 new words. This means that a common understanding not only of words but also of frame of reference between doctors and patients is difficult. 'The patient's experience of illness includes lifestyle consequences, fears and altered roles' (Keller & Carroll, 1994). For the doctor, there is a learned drivenness to arrive at the diagnosis and treat the illness.

Phenomenology

Phenomenology is the second branch or tradition of communication theory. Littlejohn & Foss (2005) state that:

> *phenomenology makes actual lived experience the basic data of*
> *reality. All you can know is what you experience. Interpretation is*
> *the process of assigning meaning to an experience; interpretation*
> *literally forms what is real for a person. When you communicate,*
> *you work out new ways of seeing the world.*

In other words, through expressing what has happened to you, you become conscious of the interpretations that you have placed on events – and what meanings you have given to them. Insight into the way that you have shaped your own reality allows meanings and interpretations to change. This process of paying attention to an individual person's lived experience in order that they may understand, change and grow is the basis of any psychotherapeutic process. Phenomenology is also fundamental to psychiatry, as history taking and mental state examination aim at hearing the patient's story and understanding what their experiences and 'symptoms' mean to them.

Beyond its relevance to the therapeutic relationship, however, phenomenology is also important in terms of the degree to which individual doctors are aware of their own interpretations and how these shape their personal ways of seeing the world. Hargie & Dickson (2004) write that 'the belief that we perceive and observe other people in a correct, factual, unbiased, objective way is a myth. Rather, what we observe typically owes as much, if not more, to ourselves in perceiving as it does to the other person in being perceived.'

Buckman (2002) writes that emotions are notoriously difficult to deal with in clinical practice: 'we may also bring our own emotional mixture to the interview: feelings in sympathy with the patient, feelings of transference, our own frustration, anger, and so on.'

Feelings of transference arise when emotion in a current situation triggers feelings from a past situation in our own personal experience, and we react to, or are affected by, the current situation in a much more emotional way than the situation actually warrants. We are not simply affected by the patient's emotion, we are experiencing and grappling with our own emotions. For example, talking to a patient about their feelings about the loss of a relative may trigger feelings that we have experienced in situations of loss, not necessarily through death, perhaps through loss of a parent in childhood through divorce, separation from a partner, loss of opportunity. The link is not always direct or obvious, and we may be defended strongly against seeing it. These issues are discussed further in Chapter 6.

In recent times, it has been increasingly recognised that, for doctors too, personal experiences and interpretations determine interpersonal reactions and influence personal styles of communication. Hargie & Dickson (2004) quote Monahan (1998) who talks of how 'interactors' evaluations of others can be influenced by non-conscious feelings derived from information sources of which they have little awareness.' Keller & Carroll (1994) suggest that it is useful for a physician to understand his or her own psychological responses to a patient, noting that Balint had explained transference and counter-transference as a method for understanding physician communication behaviours.

Countertransference in the interview situation was studied with a qualitative method among 15 medical students (Smith, 1984) and 19 residents (Smith, 1986). Some 87% and 84% respectively of these avoided psychosocial issues and /or controlled the patient excessively because of, for example, fear of hurting the patient or losing control of the situation. The students and residents were unaware of these feelings during the interview with the patient.

Cybernetics

The third contribution to communication theory comes from cybernetics, which is the study of the structure of regulatory systems. Wiener (1948) defined the term as the study of control and communication. Littlejohn & Foss (2005) discuss the family as an example of a communication system:

> *In order to understand family life, you would need to look at how the members act toward one another, how they respond to each other, how they influence one another, how they use communication to maintain stability, and how they change over time. In other words, family dynamics can only be adequately explained with a cybernetic perspective.*

Similarly, the interactions of doctors, patients, relatives, and other health care workers form a system which can be analysed and understood from a systems perspective.

Keller & Carroll (1994) write that the biomedical model was challenged by Engel's (1977) biopsychosocial model of disease:

> *He issued a call for physicians to view disease and healing as open system processes. In this new paradigm the patient becomes a systemic creature with permeable boundaries (mind/body; organism/environment) rather than a complex of isolated symptoms and physical features. Mind, body and environment are no longer separated.*

However, Maguire & Pitceathly (2002) state that doctors have been reluctant to depart from a strictly medical model. 'They have been loath to inquire about the social and emotional impact of patients' problems on the patient and family lest this unleashes distress that they cannot handle. They fear it will increase patients' distress, take up too much time, and threaten their own emotional survival.'

If the doctor does not have training in emotion handling skills, he or she may be anxious or lack confidence in seeking out patients' emotions. If the doctor avoids enquiry about social factors and emotions, the patient will find it difficult to express their feelings or the impact of the illness on his life and social functioning. The patient would like to talk more about these issues, and may feel that the doctor is uncaring and disinterested because whenever they try to tell him, the doctor changes the subject or brings the discussion back to physical symptoms. The patient may feel compelled to focus on physical issues and is not encouraged to explore the psychological meaning of some of these symptoms. The patient goes along with this, partly because they don't want to displease the doctor, and partly because he has unconscious resistance (just like the doctor) to exploring difficult psychological issues. The doctor feels comfortable they have taking control of the interview, bringing the focus back to firm ground, namely, physical and treatable symptoms, and avoiding the discomfort of not feeling confident or able to help with things which are not 'real' medical problems.

Littlejohn & Foss (2005) write that 'relationships consist of cybernetic patterns of interaction in which individuals' words and actions affect how others respond. We continually adapt our behaviours to the feedback from others, and in a relationship, both parties are doing this simultaneously.' They point out that 'power in the relationship and control within the interview is negotiated through the flow backwards and forwards of verbal messages, nonverbal signs, emotion and behaviour.'

The sociopsychological tradition

Littlejohn & Foss (2005) explain that theories in social psychology focus on:

> *individual social behaviour, psychological variables, personalities and traits, perception and cognition. They rely heavily on typing and characterizing individuals and relationships. Trait theory identifies personality variables and communicator tendencies that affect how individuals act and interact. Most sociopsychological theories of communication today are cognitive, providing insights into the way human beings process information.*

Various researchers have attempted to define distinct personality groups or types into which all people could be divided. However, this has not been particularly successful. Back in 1936, Allport and Odbert listed 18,000 descriptive words related to human personality. Cattell distilled these into 16 personality factors which were supposed to represent the basic structural elements, or building blocks, of normal personality. The 16PF personality test was widely used in the measurement of personality.

Eysenck's trait theory identified three personality factors:

1. Neuroticism: emotional stability, anxiety.
2. Extraversion: sociability and impulsivity.
3. Psychoticism: emotional warmth, aggression.

Eysenck suggested that extraverts were more sociable because they had a lower level of cortical arousal than introverts, but later studies have not consistently supported this. Psychoticism is now no longer thought to be a useful term.

Costa & McCrae (1992), in their Big Five Factor Theory, suggested five major personality traits. In addition to neuroticism and extraversion, they included agreeableness, openness to experience, and conscientiousness.

Many different personality tests and inventories have been developed. However, various problems exist with the underlying trait theories. How can a person be defined in terms of a limited number of factors? The trait approach views personality as stable through life, independent of circumstance. This is an oversimplification. Personality is not static and unchangeable, it expresses itself in different ways at different times in different circumstances. Trait theory is essentially descriptive, but has been used in an attempt to predict behaviour. However, how a person behaves in a particular situation is dependent not only on their personality but also on a number of other factors. The nature of the relationship between personality traits and behaviour has not yet been established. Most recently personality research has extended to focus on studying individual differences in affect, cognition, behaviour, experience, and learning (Boyle *et al.*, 2008).

It seems possible that personality factors may influence the ease with which doctors communicate and build relationships with different types of patients. For instance, Clack *et al.* (2004) found that doctors differed significantly from the UK adult population norms on three out of four dimensions of personality measured, and suggested that these personality differences might account for some potential points of miscommunication between doctors and patients. They used the Myers-Briggs Type Indicator (MBTI), a popular personality test which places an individual in one of sixteen types, some people overlapping two or three types. It uses Carl Jung's classifications of introversion and extraversion, and his descriptions of the four functions of sensing, thinking, intuition and feeling, which are developed to varying degrees in different people.

According to the MBTI, my (TP) results are INTJ (introverted intuiting with thinking). The description is as follows: 'These are the most independent of all types. They love logic and ideas and are drawn to scientific research. They can be rather single-minded, though.' Like horoscopes, some bits fit and some don't.

Other researchers, rather than looking at personality factors, have focused on the characteristics or behaviours that doctors might be expected to exhibit in the doctor-patient interaction. For example, in a study of 215 patients, Beach *et al.* (2006) found that doctors strongly agreed that they had a great deal of respect for 34% of patients, agreed for 45% of patients and were either neutral or disagreed for 21% of patients. Doctors reported higher levels of respect for older patients and for patients they knew well; they provided more information and expressed more positive affect to those patients. The level of respect was primarily associated with familiarity rather than sociodemographic characteristics such as gender, race, education or health status.

It is interesting to speculate on the reasons why the levels of respect varied so much. It may be that the doctors had grown to know and like certain patients over a period of time, and were perhaps less anxious themselves about the consultations because they already had a relationship and knowledge of the patient's problems. Consequently, they were able to talk more and show more positive feelings.

Irwin & Richardson (2006) quote a survey of 157 adolescent female patients (aged 14 to 19 years) who were asked to describe the ideal physician. They found that:

> *87% of the "ideal" characteristics identified related to communication. Medical behaviour determined only 10% of wanted characteristics. Within the theme of communication, "understanding" (18%) and "talks to me" (15%) were the most important characteristics, followed by "cares" (10%), "listens" (8%), and "respect" (7%). For this age group, high-quality communication and a focus on them as a person were important needs.*

Berry (2007) makes the point that 'doctors and patients have very different views on the most important quality of a good doctor,' and quotes Paling (2004) who found that 'for doctors, it is diagnostic ability, whereas for patients it is listening. Doctors rated listening as least important.' Keller & Carroll (1994) found that in order for doctors to rate health care as excellent, it must be firstly technically excellent and secondly, the doctor must be empathic and present to the patient as a human being.

Chapter 3

The sociocultural tradition
Littlejohn & Foss (2005) state that:

> *the sociocultural tradition attempts to understand ways in which people together create the realities of their social groups, organisations and cultures. People use language differently in different social and cultural groups. Identity is negotiated from one situation to another. The sociocultural tradition has been influenced by ethnomethodology, which influences how we look at conversations, including the way in which participants manage the back-and-forth flow with language and nonverbal behaviours.*

Roter *et al.* (2002) found that primary care consultations with female doctors were, on average, two minutes (10%) longer than those with male doctors. There were no gender differences in the amount, quality, or manner of biomedical information giving or social conversation. However, female physicians engaged in significantly more active partnership behaviours, positive talk, psychosocial counselling, psychosocial question asking, and emotionally focused talk. They point out that in obstetrics and gynaecology, however, male physicians demonstrate higher levels of emotionally focused talk than their female colleagues.

Hall & Roter (2002), in a meta-analysis of seven observational studies, found that overall, 'patients spoke more to female physicians than to male physicians, disclosed more biomedical and psychosocial information and made more positive statements to female physicians. Patients also rated as more assertive toward female physicians and tended to interrupt them more.'

Ferguson & Candib's review (2002) found evidence that 'race, ethnicity, and language have substantial influence on the quality of the doctor-patient relationship. Minority patients, especially those not proficient in English, are less likely to engender empathic response from physicians, establish rapport with physicians, receive sufficient information, and be encouraged to participate in medical decision making.' Furthermore, Kaplan *et al.* (1996) found that non-white physicians were reported by patients to be less participatory than white physicians.

A study by Ohtaki *et al.* (2003) compared consultations in the US and Japan, and found that the US physicians spent relatively more time on treatment and follow-up talk and social talk, whereas the Japanese had longer physical examinations and diagnosis or consideration talk. Notable cultural differences included longer silences/pauses during Japanese encounters, which give more time for the listener to consider the speaker's feelings and thoughts.

The critical tradition

Littlejohn & Foss (2005) state that the critical tradition 'explores the questions of privilege and power in communication theory. It shows that power, oppression, and privilege are the products of certain forms of communication throughout society.' They explain that the language used by dominant or powerful people can have the effect of marginalising less powerful people because the latter are less able or unable to use or understand that language.

Charles *et al.* (2000) write that 'the voice of medicine is characterised by medical terminology, objective descriptions, and classifications within a biomedical model. The voice of patients on the other hand is characterised by non-technical discourse about the subjective experience of illness within the context of social relationships and the patient's everyday world.' Waitzkin's view (1984) is that doctors often maintain a style of high control, which involves many doctor-initiated questions, interruptions, and neglect of patients' 'life world.'

Keller & Carroll (1994) suggest that the physician-patient relationship can be viewed as a consequence of how each behaves at a verbal level, or of the roles they play. The doctor's contribution to the dialogue depends both on their communication skills repertoire, and on the psychological difficulties and strengths that they bring to the interaction. They quote Emanuel and Emanuel (1992) who describe 'four role possibilities for the physician to enact: paternalistic, informative, interpretive, and deliberative.'

Skelton & Hobbs (1999) conducted an analysis of the doctor-patient consultation in primary care using computer concordancing, a methodology used in linguistic research to study both the quantitative and qualitative aspects of language. They analysed the language of 40 doctors and their patients during 373 consultations, looking at 'the use of jargon by doctors, the language of power and absence of power, and ways in which language was used to diminish the potential threat of the presenting disorder.'

They found that although the doctors did not use medical jargon, this did not mean that they were easily understood:

> *some doctors used language associated with social power, and some patients used language associated with absence of power, which could mean that their consultations were less democratic than they should be. Doctors frequently used language to express emotions (eg anxiety), to diminish threats (eg words such as "little"), and to reassure patients, which was interpreted as denoting a therapeutic use of language.*

The rhetorical tradition

Littlejohn & Foss (2005) believe that the communication discipline began with rhetoric, which, broadly defined, is human symbol use: 'Originally concerned with persuasion, rhetoric was the art of constructing arguments and speechmaking. The focus of rhetoric has now broadened to encompass all of the ways humans use symbols to affect those around them and to construct the worlds in which they live.'

An interesting study was conducted by Pennebaker & Francis (1996) in which college students were asked to write either about their thoughts and feelings about coming to college or about superficial topics for three consecutive days. They found that writing about upsetting experiences was found to reduce health centre visits for illness and to improve subjects' grade point average. Text analyses indicated that the use of positive emotion words and changes in words suggestive of causal and insightful thinking were linked to health change.

In other words, there is a purpose to communication which goes far beyond the conveying of information. When we think or write, we are communicating with ourselves. When we talk to others, we are in addition also communicating with ourselves. Through articulating our thoughts and feelings, we bring them to consciousness, we re-examine and redefine attitudes and emotions. In other words, through communication, we actually change our minds. Which was the whole point of rhetoric in the first place.

Verbal and nonverbal communication

We all have varying degrees of conscious awareness of how we communicate and interact with others. 'Nonverbal behaviour provides a great deal of information very quickly (Ambady & Rosenthal, 1993), yet people are often unaware of their own and others' nonverbal behaviour' (Hall *et al.*, 1995). We communicate information in many different ways all at the same time: about the topic of discussion; about ourselves, our feelings, our world view, our mood at that moment – and our reactions to the other person. Every human interaction is a complex interplay of actions and reactions. We emit signals – physically, energetically, emotionally, and verbally, as soon as we encounter another person – and we sense and receive responses.

Hall *et al.* (1995) state that 'the two-way flow of nonverbal cues between provider and patient is now recognised as highly important in medical training and medical practice (Lipkin, Quill & Napodano, 1984; Novack *et al.*, 1993; Roter & Hall, 1992; Simpson *et al.*, 1991; Zinn, 1993).' The Royal College of Physicians report (1997) points out that 'doctors need to be sensitive to the non-verbal behaviour of patients as well as be aware that their own non-verbal communication may convey negative messages.'

As far back as 1979, Friedman described the role of sensitivity and expressiveness in both the patient and the clinician (Hall *et al.*, 1995). DiMatteo *et al.* (1986) describe these two dimensions of nonverbal communication:

> *(a) decoding or sensitivity and (b) encoding or expressiveness. Nonverbal decoding refers to the capacity to understand the emotions conveyed through others' nonverbal cues such as facial expressions, body movements and voice tone. Nonverbal encoding refers to the capacity to express emotion through nonverbal cues.*

In other words, decoding is being able to pick up on other people's emotions. Bull (2001) states that 'six emotions have been shown to be decoded in the same way by members of both literate and pre-literate cultures – happiness, sadness, anger, fear, disgust, surprise – and a possible seventh is contempt.'

Being observant, we can gather a great deal of important information. When we meet a person, we notice their appearance, and their mood – we know if they are angry, or upset about something. Within the first seconds, we take in details of their clothing, their facial appearance, the way they hold themselves, the way they shake hands, and we listen to them talking. We observe their facial expressions, eye contact and body posture as they speak. In the therapeutic relationship, it is important to be able to sense how a person feels, and to respond to their emotional cues. 'The patient's nonverbal behaviour (for example, sighs, voice qualities and pitch, posture, brimming of the eyes) can call our attention to emotionally charged material' (Heath, 1984). If the doctor is not sensitive, the patient may never be able to say what is troubling him. It is very helpful to explore patients' feelings, as these may influence their relationship with the doctor, their engagement with treatment, their reactions to their illness, and their level of satisfaction.

DiMatteo *et al.* (1980) studied internal medicine residents interacting with their patients in order to investigate the relationship between doctors' nonverbal communication skills (their ability to communicate and to understand facial expression, body movement and voice tone cues to emotion) and their patients' satisfaction with medical care. They found that:

> *nonverbal communication skills bore little relationship to patients' ratings of technical quality of care, but measures of nonverbal skills did predict patient satisfaction with the art of medical care received. Doctors who were more sensitive to body movement and posture cues to emotion (the channel suggested by nonverbal researchers as the one in which true affect can be perceived) received higher ratings from their patients on the art of care than did less sensitive physicians.*

Encoding or expressiveness is the other part of nonverbal communication. People vary a great deal in how much eye contact they use, their posture, how much they smile, or reassure, or react emotionally to the other person's expressed emotion. People also vary in the extent of their self-awareness, the degree to which they are conscious of the signals that they give out about their level of interest, mood, feelings, or supposedly private thoughts.

Roter *et al.* (2002) state that:

> *nonverbal communication includes positive nonverbal behaviours (smiles, nods, friendly voice tone, relaxed hands), and a variety of behaviours that can have ambiguous, neutral, or negative meaning depending on the context of use (eg touches patient, folds hands, gestures while speaking, points at the patient, speech is disturbed, voice tone reflects anxiety or boredom).*

They conducted a meta-analysis of 26 studies, mostly in primary care, of gender effects in medical communication. 'Of six which assessed positive nonverbal behaviour, two reported significant results showing that female physicians demonstrate higher levels of smiling and head nods (Hall *et al.*, 1994), and awareness of nonverbal communication (Shapiro, 1990). No studies reported higher levels of positive nonverbal behaviour for male physicians.'

However, Mast *et al.* (2008) point out that, to be satisfied, patients expect female and male physicians to show different patterns of nonverbal behaviour. Their study found that patients were most satisfied with female physicians who behaved in line with the female gender role (eg more gazing, more forward lean, softer voice) while still stressing their professionalism (medical-looking examination room). For male physicians, satisfaction was high for a broader range of behaviours, partly related to their gender role (eg louder voice, more distance to patient).

Larsen & Smith (1981) draw attention to two major nonverbal categories, immediacy and relaxation. Hall *et al.* (1995) describe immediacy as 'behaviours that describe a positive involved relation between interactants, including such cues as close proximity, forward lean, open arm and leg postures, facing one another, eye contact and postural relaxation (Anderson, 1985; Mehrabian, 1972).' Hall *et al.* (1995) report a number of studies which showed that:

> *the most important cues for expressing empathy, genuineness and respect were forward trunk lean, close distance and eye contact (Haase & Tepper, 1972; Hermansson et al. 1988; Tepper & Haase,*

1978). Harrigan et al. (1985) have demonstrated that doctors who face their patients directly, make more eye contact and maintain open arm postures are regarded as more empathic, interested and warm.

Platt *et al.* (2001) state that 'undivided attention is the strongest evidence of a desire to help the patient. Leaning slightly toward the patient, nodding, making eye contact, and using facilitative hums and murmurs all show interest.'

Hall & Roter (2002) state that 'behaviours such as gazing, smiling, posture, a variety of speech behaviours and the emotional tone of one's communication are typically reciprocated or matched in social interactions.' This can be assessed by untrained observers from video clips ranging from a few seconds to a few minutes. Hall *et al.* (1995) point out that when good rapport is established, this matching reaches the level of synchronisation. Interactional synchrony is said to occur when the rhythm established between people as they interact is coordinated and smooth, their postures and movements occur simultaneously and intertwine.

Hall *et al.* (1995) state that relating to patients through expressive nonverbal cues appears to be an essential skill for the physician. DiMatteo *et al.* (1980) found that doctors who were successful at expressing emotion through their nonverbal communications tended to receive higher ratings from patients on the art of care than did physicians who were less effective communicators. In 1986, DiMatteo *et al.* again showed that nonverbal encoding skill was significantly related to patient satisfaction. However, several other studies have found no association of patient satisfaction with various nonverbal behaviours (Griffiths *et al.*, 2003).

Tate (2007) pointed out that 'looking at video recordings of consultations, it is surprising how often doctors do not seem to be very interested in their patient as an individual.' Heath (1984) found that patients use gestures to try to regain eye contact if the doctor has looked away. Ruusuvuori (2001) found that patients find it problematic when doctors start reading or writing in the medical records, as they are not sure whether the doctor is still listening. Hall *et al.* (1995) quoted a study by Duncan *et al.* (1968) which showed that, in peak hours, psychotherapists sounded serious, warm and relaxed, whereas during poor hours, their voices sounded dull, flat and uninvolved.

Hall *et al.* (1995) state that:

> *rapport and empathy are built when behaviours include attentive listening and not talking too much, avoiding excessive note taking and chart reading, establishing eye contact, leaning forward, establishing an appropriate interpersonal distance, encouraging the patient to speak by using facilitators such as smiles, nods and "uh huh" responses and showing affect.*

Platt *et al.* (2001) state that 'to be truly patient-centred, physicians must demonstrate both verbally and nonverbally that the most important part of the medical interview is the person facing them.' Indeed, as Bull (2001) points out, 'nonverbal cues appear to be more important than speech in judgements of rapport. Nonverbal communication has sometimes been regarded as a kind of language of emotion and interpersonal relationships.'

Hargie & Dickson (2004) write that:

> *the nonverbal channel of communication is frequently more important than the verbal channel with regard to the conveying of information of an emotional or attitudinal nature. Indeed, when information of this type resulting from one channel contradicts that carried by means of the other, greater credence is often placed on the nonverbal message. It would, therefore, seem that the nonverbal channel is particularly adept at communicating states and attitudes such as friendliness, interest, warmth and involvement.*

A frequently quoted study conducted by Mehrabian in 1972 estimated that overall communication is made up of body language (55%), paralanguage (the nonverbal aspects of speech) 38% and the verbal 7% – but this only applies when verbal and nonverbal information are non-congruent. In other words, if the verbal message is being contradicted by the nonverbal message, then the nonverbal message carries most weight. For instance, if I say, 'Hello, I'm really pleased to see you,' and I am frowning, talking in an unenthusiastic tone of voice, and walking away from you, then unsurprisingly, you won't feel very welcome, and you won't believe what I am saying.

If, on the other hand, I walk towards you, smiling, holding out my hand and saying excitedly, 'Hello, I'm really pleased to see you,' then the information is congruent; in other words that from the verbal channel supports and reinforces that from nonverbal channels, and the contribution of the verbal communication is far more than 7%.

Mehrabian's study is often misquoted as this distinction is not made, and the impression is created that verbal communication is always less important than nonverbal, which is clearly untrue. As Hargie & Dickson (2004) report, 'these proportions seriously under-represent the contribution of verbal communication in circumstances where information from all three channels is largely congruent.' They quote Burgoon *et al.* (1996) who identified 'a general trend favouring the primacy of meaning carried nonverbally, with a reliance on visual cues, particularly for adults, in situations of message incongruity and where the message has to do with emotional, relational or impression-forming outcomes.'

Griffiths *et al.* (2003) state that 'nonverbal communication is intimately related to verbal communication; it often anticipates, substitutes for, augments, accentuates, or, importantly, contradicts verbal communication and is a primary vehicle for expressing emotion.' They quote Nardone *et al.* (1992) who write that nonverbal cues 'may be less susceptible to censorship than verbal cues and therefore may be more reliable indicators of what is being communicated.' Hargie & Dickson (2004) report that nonverbal communication can be thought of as 'a more "truthful" form of communication through the insights that it affords into what may lie behind the verbal message,' although they warn against hard and fast rules as social context can clearly influence facial displays of emotion. Hall *et al.* (1995) report that 'inconsistent cues from counsellor verbal and nonverbal channels produce negative evaluations,' and they quote Graves & Robinson (1976) who found that counsellors who gave inconsistent messages were perceived as less genuine and caused clients to react by increasing their distance from the counsellor.

A quite astonishing American article by Larson & Yao (2005) proposes 'that physicians consider empathy as emotional labor – management of experienced and displayed emotions to present a certain image.' They urge doctors 'to engage in such emotional labor either through surface acting, in which individuals can fake their emotional display by forging facial expressions, voice, or posture or through deep acting, in which they can try to alter their internal experience and act on emotions they actually experience.'

They report that the concept of emotional labor, the 'act of expressing organizationally desired emotions during service transactions,' is well-known in organizational management, for instance it has been used with flight attendants and bill collectors – 'but it is not widely appreciated in medicine.' Thank goodness for that!

It is our belief that doctors generally strive to be honest and genuine in their relationships and interactions with patients. As Stewart (2005) says:

> *this relationship requires an openness on the part of the doctor to learning about all of the dimensions of a patient's problems – and a willingness to meet the patient at an emotional level not only in order to have an understanding of the problems, but also to facilitate a healing of the whole person. This way of being a doctor requires engaging at both the cognitive level and the emotional level, but also tapping into a doctor's intuition, the creative side which puts together complex webs of different types of information (cognitive, emotional and intuitive) into a new insight, not singly but with the patient.*

Communication skills training

It is thought that in a forty-year career a doctor will conduct between 150,000 and 200,000 interviews with patients and their families. And, as Langewitz *et al.* (1998) point out, 'it can be assumed that clinical experience per se does improve some communication skills, specifically those related to the identification of medical information and those related to the communication of treatment options.' These are relatively basic communication tasks. However, other more complex aspects of communication do not necessarily improve simply with repeating old habits. Fallowfield *et al.* (2002) state that very few doctors have received much formal training in communication, and the training provided is commonly inadequate.

Feinmann (2002) quotes Ong who states that:

> *certain specialties are particularly demanding in testing doctors'*
> *ability to communicate. Paediatricians have to communicate*
> *effectively and empathetically with children – from babies to 18*
> *year olds – as well as with very worried and demanding parents.*
> *A gynaecologist's consultation may well cover sexuality, sexual*
> *abuse, pregnancy, childbirth, menopause, or cancer. And in a single*
> *consultation, oncologists, surgeons, and intensive care doctors*
> *have, on a regular basis, to tell families that the patient has died*
> *and discuss a post-mortem and organ donation.*

Yet Feinmann (2002) reports that, 'given the option to attend a communication skills course, many doctors decline, especially surgeons, who are among those most resistant to acknowledging the need to brush up their talking skills.'

According to Tate (2007):

> *the problem as shown by experience and research work is that*
> *doctors do not change. Audio and visual recordings of multiple*
> *consultations by the same doctor show a remarkable consistency*
> *of style. Doctors say and do things in much the same way with an*
> *anxious 16 year old coming for a termination as with a 50-year old*
> *woman with menorrhagia or an 80-year old woman with vulval*
> *carcinoma. It appears that we do not regularly adapt to meet the*
> *needs of the patient. We need to be flexible, and it appears that*
> *most of us are not.*

Communication training is still developing (Buckman, 2002). Various studies have shown that communication skills training courses lasting one day or less are not effective (Aspegren, 1999), and that longer courses are more effective, for example Jenkins & Fallowfield (2002) report that clinicians who attended a 3-day course demonstrated and maintained improvements in communication skills over those who attended a 1.5-day course. Aspegren (1999) stated that 'the teaching method should be experiential as it has been shown conclusively that instructional methods do not give desired results. The content of communication skills courses should primarily be problem defining. Men are slower learners of communication skills than women, which should be taken into account by course organizers.' Rees & Sheard (2002) quote a number of researchers who have suggested that 'lecture-based teaching is less effective in terms of communication skills learning than more practically oriented and problem-based learning.' Aspegren (1999) points out that skills are forgotten if not practised, and quotes Pfeiffer *et al.* (1999) who found that acquired skills often decline.

For undergraduate courses, Hargie *et al.* (1998) found that there is considerable variability in course content, timing, duration and methods of assessment. Cegala & Broz (2002) point out that most medical schools now include some form of communication instruction in their curriculum, although Hulsman *et al.* (1999) did note that the actual time devoted to it may be minimal. Hargie *et al.* (1998) conducted a survey of UK medical schools and found that:

> *the student could receive a total of between 3 and 16 communication skills training sessions throughout the duration of the medical course (theoretical sessions lasted between 40 minutes and 2 hours, and practical sessions ranged between 1 and 3 hours). In all schools, tuition was offered by the Department of General Practice, with the next most frequent being psychiatry. Theoretical components included attitude theory, social interaction, the psychology of group behaviour and group dynamics, cognitive aspects of communication, compliance, and medical ethics. The main communication skills taught included breaking bad news, information giving, information gathering, counselling, interviewing, assertiveness and negotiation, and written skills.*

Buyck & Lang (2002) reported that:

> *faculty of medical education programs who teach communications varied widely in identifying teachable moments across all six communication categories: rapport building, agenda setting, information management, active listening for the patient's perspective, responding to emotion, and skills in reaching common ground. For instance, of 67 respondents, 29.6% identified none of the opportunities to teach rapport building, while only 31% identified all opportunities.*

Staff factors found in Hargie *et al.*'s survey (1998) included lack of suitably trained staff; lack of CST experience and overt opposition to

CST; cost of simulated patients; and lack of suitable accommodation. Staff training was anticipated to range from two days to two hours across schools.

Kinnersley & Spencer (2008) write that 'it is only recently that we have moved from the belief that entrants to medical school, by virtue of their intelligence, are innately effective and sensitive communicators, and that any who aren't can pick up the skills by osmosis and good intentions.' The UK Council for Communication Skills Teaching in Undergraduate Medical Education (von Fragstein *et al.*, 2008) has produced a consensus statement on the key content of communication curricula.

A central component of this statement is the communication curriculum wheel, in which the key domains are shown as concentric rings, starting in the centre with 'respect for others.'

Tasks outlined in the consensus statement (von Fragstein *et al.*, 2008) include:

- Establishing and building a relationship.
- Initiating (ie opening the consultation and seeing the agenda).
- Establishing, recognising and meeting patients' needs.
- Gathering information.
- Eliciting and considering the patient's world views.
- Conducting a physical examination.
- Formulating and explaining relevant diagnoses.
- Explaining, planning and negotiating.
- Structuring, signposting and prioritising, and
- Closing (ending the interview and setting up the next meeting).

Skills outlined in the consensus statement (von Fragstein *et al.*, 2008) include:

- Eye contact.
- Facial expression.
- Attentive listening.
- Screening.
- Appropriate balance of open and closed questions.

- Facilitation.
- Empathic reflection.
- Responding to cues (both verbal and non-verbal).
- Summarising.
- Signposting.
- Determining the patient's starting point when giving information.
- Chunking information, and
- Checking the patient's understanding.

Efficacy of communication skills training

Nineteen studies of communication skills training showed that medical students improved their ability to interview and/or gain information from patients after attending such courses (Sanson-Fisher & Poole, 1978). Evans *et al.* (1991) showed that after training, 'students had improved interviewing skills and interpersonal effectiveness, and were diagnostically more efficient without taking longer to elicit the information.' However, Rees & Sheard (2002) found that 'students with more negative attitudes towards communication skills learning tended to think their communication skills did not need improving.' Their study showed that women students had more positive attitudes towards communication skills learning. Students whose first language was not English, and those whose ethnicity was non-white scored significantly higher on negative attitudes towards communication skills learning. Maguire *et al.* (1977) found that in general, when students' self rating of their communication skills has been compared with external independent rating there is a low correlation.

It does not seem sufficient merely to teach communication skills at medical school – postgraduate courses are also required. Cegala & Broz (2002) identified 26 studies of doctor communication skills training between 1990 and 2002 from both sides of the Atlantic. 'The majority of studies included insufficient information about the communication behaviours taught to participants. In several studies there was a mismatch between stated behaviours and instruments or procedures used to assess them.' They reported little consistency in what is considered to be a communication skill, and little effort to provide a framework for communication skills. Griffin *et al.* (2004) identified 35 trials in the US, mainly in primary care, up to the end of 1999. Studies tended to be small and short with major design limitations. 'Interventions frequently combined several poorly described elements. Explicit theoretical underpinning was rare, and only one study linked intervention through process to outcome measures. Health outcomes were rarely measured objectively (6 out of 35), and only 4 trials with health outcomes met predefined quality criteria.' The authors concluded that collection of better evidence is required to inform practice.

It has been suggested that competence in communication consists of motivation, knowledge and social skill (Spitzberg, 1983); it requires both effectiveness and appropriateness of communication (Mizco et al., 2001). Various researchers have expressed concerns related to the effectiveness and appropriateness of communication skills training courses. Aspegren (1999) quotes Cooper & Mira (1998) who state that 'communication skills emphasized by academic teachers do not reflect the skills considered important by patients.' Betz Brown et al. (1999) found that training did not improve patient satisfaction scores: they suggested that 'to improve global visit satisfaction, communication skills training programs may need to be longer and more intensive, teach a broader range of skills, and provide ongoing performance feedback.'

Kinnersley et al. (2008) noted that training clinicians can be expensive and may not improve performance or other outcomes. Skelton & Hobbs (1999) state that 'many quantitative studies presume that interaction can be reduced to the counting of behaviours, for instance, deconstructing consultations into discrete points, defined in behavioural (and therefore observable) terms that boost test reliability – for example, did the doctor greet the patient; were open questions asked?' Kidd et al. (2005) report that 'the current practice of teaching communication skills separately from clinical skills reflects a reductionist paradigm – by breaking down the complex phenomenon of a consultation to its basic components. This limits coherence and leads to unbalanced doctors.' They suggest that learning communication and clinical skills side by side would be more effective.

Aspegren (1999) claims that 'there is overwhelming evidence for a positive effect of communication skills training (Rutter & Maguire 1976; Maguire et al., 1977),' yet Shilling et al. (2003) report that studies that have examined the effects of training on patient and doctors' satisfaction have produced equivocal findings. Like Hulsman *et al.* (2002), they found no significant increase in patient satisfaction as a result of clinician communication skills training. However, Langewitz *et al.* (1998) make the point that intervention programs up till then had used quite different outcome measures: these include patient satisfaction scores, psychiatric knowledge, self-assessed competence, or linguistic discourse characteristics. For example, Joos *et al.* (1996) trained doctors in eliciting and responding to patients' concerns and requests, and found that they improved in both of these areas compared with controls. However, the intervention was not associated with changes in patient compliance with medications or appointments, nor were there any effects on outpatient utilization.

A systematic review by Lewin *et al.* (2001) found 17 trials of training interventions designed to promote a more patient-centred approach in clinical consultations. They found that:

> *there is fairly strong evidence to suggest that some interventions to promote patient-centred care may lead to significant increases in the patient-centredness of consultation processes, as indicated by a range of measures relating to clarifying patients' concerns and beliefs; communicating about treatment options; levels of empathy etc. Of the eleven studies that assessed patient satisfaction, six demonstrated significant differences in favour of the intervention group on one or more measures.*

The authors concluded that it is difficult to quantify the benefits or effects of training, and therefore difficult to give recommendations to policy makers and professional bodies regarding investment into the development of such training. They drew attention to the need to develop a widely acceptable definition of patient-centred care.

How are skills learned?

Hargie & Dickson (2004) characterise skilled performance as:

- Controlled by the individual.
- Learned behaviour that improves with practice and feedback.

- Integrated and interrelated verbal and nonverbal responses.
- Purposive and goal-directed.
- Smooth in the manner in which the performance is executed.

According to Maguire & Pitceathly (2002), effective teaching methods should:

- Provide evidence of current deficiencies in communication, reasons for them, and the consequences for patients and doctors.
- Offer an evidence base for the skills needed to overcome these deficiencies.
- Demonstrate the skills to be learned and elicit reactions to these.
- Provide an opportunity to practise the skills under controlled and safe conditions.
- Give constructive feedback on performance and reflect on the reasons for any blocking behaviour.

Maguire & Pitceathly (2002) suggest that communication skills training should include three components of learning: cognitive input, modelling, and practice of key skills. These three categories will be examined in greater depth below.

Cognitive input

This includes education, discussion, and the examination and challenging of beliefs that may be restricting or limiting the possibilities for change. It may involve reframing of the problem to be able to begin to solve it in a different way. For example, Levinson *et al.* (1993) conducted a workshop with 1,076 doctors from multiple specialties, in which 'frustrating' visits were explored with a view to developing a guide to help doctors identify the cause of problems in communicating with patients. They found that doctors most often attributed communication problems to the patient rather than to their own limitations. Seven types of communication problems were identified: 1) lack of trust / agreement, 2) too many problems, 3) feeling distressed, 4) lack of understanding, 5) lack of adherence, 6) demanding/controlling patient, and 7) special problems.

Fallowfield *et al.* (2002) conducted a randomised controlled trial to assess the efficacy of an intensive 3-day training course on communication skills for 160 oncologists. Following the course, which involved structured feedback, videotape review, role-play with simulated patients, interactive group demonstrations, and discussion led by a trained facilitator, doctors reported a greater degree of confidence when dealing with difficult communication problems. They also showed improved communication skills in clinic consultations compared with controls. The changes included a reduction in closed, leading questions, an increase in open and focused questions, more appropriate responses to patients' cues, and more empathic responses.

Jenkins & Fallowfield (2002) make the point that 'doctors who engage in patient-centred behaviour should not only demonstrate good communication skills and actively probe patients' psychosocial concerns, but they should also exhibit positive beliefs and attitudes toward the importance of such behaviours.' They quote Levinson and Roter (1995), who used an adaptation of the Physician Psychosocial Belief (PPSB) scale with primary care doctors. They found that those who had positive scores on the psychosocial belief scale used more statements expressing emotion and empathy in their consultations and provided patients with more psychosocial and less biomedical information than physicians with less positive attitudes. In addition, the patients of these doctors expressed more opinions and asked more questions.

Jenkins & Fallowfield (2002) also used the Physician Psychosocial Belief scale with 93 oncologists. Those who attended a 3-day residential communication skills course showed significantly improved attitudes and beliefs toward psychosocial issues compared with controls, and this was reflected in video analysis of their consultations. Expressions of empathy were more likely, as were open questions, appropriate responses to patient cues, and psychosocial probing.

The communication skills training intervention used behavioural, cognitive, and affective components, and it was the view of the researchers that all three of these components may be necessary to produce change. The training not only led to more effective interviewing styles, but can also alter attitudes and beliefs, thus increasing the likelihood that such skills will be used in the clinical setting.

Modelling

Langewitz *et al.* (1998) taught a behaviourally oriented intervention to residents in Internal Medicine for 22.5 hours over a 6-month period. They found that it was useful for participants to see themselves in video feedback; to try alternative behaviours once the problem had been identified; and to define individual goals after the workshop. They noted that trying alternative behaviour often elicited uncomfortable feelings in the physician and in those watching, but they felt that being in the patients' position in role play was crucial.

Practice of key skills

It appears that doctors find it difficult to transfer learned skills and behaviours into clinical practice (Langewitz *et al.*, 1998; Maguire & Pitceathly, 2002). Individual skills need to be practised until they can be comfortably and effectively used. Two examples given by Langewitz *et al.* (1998) are negotiating and taking up emotions. They suggested that doctors offer a negotiating process during the interview, for example by announcing explicitly a change in the topic and the structure of the communication. This orientates the patient, for instance: 'Thank you for explaining your concerns, I think I have quite a clear idea of what has been happening for you recently. I would now like to shift focus to ask some specific questions about your symptoms, then we'll have some time to discuss options about treatment.' Langewitz *et al.* (2002) showed that doctors 'can learn to listen actively to patients, to invite the patient to share decisions, and to negotiate about the process of health care.'

Langewitz *et al.* (1998) described taking up emotions as a specific skill requiring practice. It is clearly a key area for improvement for many doctors. Roter & Hall (1995) state that 'despite high prevalence, emotional distress among primary care patients often goes unrecognized during routine medical encounters.' Jenkins & Fallowfield (2002) also comment that 'many physicians worldwide working within oncology fail to identify their patients' distress. They do not actively probe psychological problems because of poor communication skills, apprehension about dealing with emotional issues, or a belief that such areas are not part of their remit.'

Roter *et al.* (1995) found that important changes in doctors' communication skills were evident after an 8-hour training course designed to help doctors address patients' emotional distress through problem-defining and emotion-handling skills. They found that:

> *the training improved the process and outcome of care without lengthening the visits. Trained physicians used significantly more problem-defining and emotion-handling skills than did untrained physicians; they reported more psychosocial problems, engaged in more strategies for managing emotional problems in actual patients, and scored higher in clinical proficiency with simulated patients. Patients of trained physicians reported reduction in emotional distress for as long as 6 months.*

Other studies have also shown that patients benefit from doctors' ability to deal with emotional issues. For instance, Shilling *et al.* (2003) quote studies showing that 'patients who perceive the clinicians' behaviour in the diagnostic consultation as being "caring" or "emotionally supportive" have better psychological adjustment both in the short (Roberts *et al.*, 1994) and long term (Mager & Andrykowski, 2002).'

Haskard *et al.* (2008) report that communication skills training for doctors improved patients' satisfaction with 'information and overall care; increased physicians' counselling (as reported by patients) about weight loss, exercise, and quitting smoking and alcohol; and increased independent ratings of physicians' sensitive, connected communication with their patients.'

Chapter 4

Communication skills

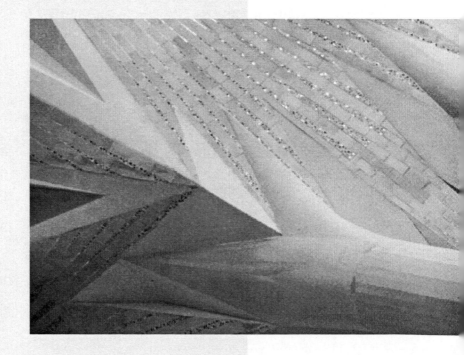

Communication skills

In the last chapter, various models were described which explore the contribution of different fields of knowledge and research to the development of a body of information about communication. Models provide a theoretical framework. They stimulate thought and discussion, and they help us to understand a subject with greater depth and complexity. When a model is in place, we then need a structure, a practical way of applying theory. A conceptual understanding needs to be supported by guidelines for skilful application.

This chapter looks at a number of ways of structuring the medical interview with a view to highlighting the specific communication skills required at each step. However, when a structure has been decided, models learned, and theories taken into consideration, we are still on our own. In the consulting room. Communicating. If we merely take a formulaic approach, this can threaten to turn what essentially is a dynamic, fluid, constantly changing system into something static and repetitive. Furthermore, there simply is not the time to work through yet another long list of questions. We must develop the capacity to be creative. We can use communication skills learning in combination with day-to-day clinical experience to try out new ways of interacting. This is an iterative process in which experiential learning feeds back into our theoretical understanding and influences our beliefs about what communication actually involves and how it works.

In terms of consultation tasks, Cegala & Broz (2002) state that 'some scholars have suggested a classification following a distinction between information exchange and relational development (Sanson-Fisher & Cockburn, 1997) while others have organised skills according to the stage, or component, of the medical interview (Silverman *et al.*, 1998).' Either way, certain tasks have to be achieved in the consultation within the context of the doctor-patient relationship.

The degree of patient-centredness seems to be a measure of certain components of communication. Little *et al.* (2001a) stated that 'from the patients' perspective there are probably at least three important and distinct domains of patient-centredness: communication, partnership, and health promotion.' Irwin & Richardson (2006) confirm that these areas constitute patient-focused care, in addition to the physical care, medications and treatments provided. They write of the 'three Cs' – communication, continuity of care, and concordance (finding common ground).

Campion *et al.* (2002) quote Mead & Bower (2000) who state that 'patient centeredness comprises five dimensions: a biopsychosocial perspective, the patient-as-person, sharing power and responsibility, the therapeutic alliance, and the doctor-as-person.'

Campion *et al.* (2002) assessed 2094 candidates on video consultations for the Member of the Royal College of General Practitioners, (MRCGP) exam. They found that 69% of candidates met the criteria in at least three of five consultations; they encouraged the patient's contribution, obtained information, carried out appropriate examination, made the diagnosis and explained it in appropriate language, made a management plan, prescribed appropriately, and achieved rapport. Six criteria measured aspects of patient-centredness: not ignoring cues, exploring social and psychological content, exploring health understanding, explanation taking account of patient's beliefs, confirming patient's understanding of the explanation, and sharing management options. Only 36% managed to involve patients in decision-making. They concluded that:

> doctors nearing completion of a three year postgraduate training in general practice showed only limited ability to achieve patient-centred outcomes. The ability to elicit patients' ideas, concerns, and expectations is fundamental to good consulting, but our results suggest that few doctors regularly use this ability, even in a highly selected set of consultations. Likewise, the checking of understanding and the involving of patients in decision making – both likely to improve concordance – are rarely demonstrated.

The report of the Royal College of Physicians (1997) presents a model modified from Morris & Schofield (1992) which provides a checklist of steps needed for a successful and satisfying consultation:

1. Relationship: establishes an effective relationship with the patient and demonstrates respect for the patient as a person.
2. Structuring: conducts the consultation in a sequence logical to that particular patient's needs, and lets the patient know and follow the sequence, so that time is used effectively.
3. History: elicits the patient's history and symptoms, their chronology and related factors, sufficiently to establish their possible causes.
4. Question style: demonstrates the appropriate use of open, closed and reflective questions.
5. Listening: listens to the patient and responds to cues.
6. Patient's understanding and ideas: explores the patient's understanding and ideas about the nature and cause of the problems and their management.
7. Patient's worries and concerns: explores and responds to the patient's worries and concerns about the problems and their management.
8. Explaining: offers the patient an appropriate explanation of the problems and their management which is related to the patient's own ideas.
9. Checking: checks that the patient understands any explanations and that concerns have been addressed.
10. Involving: takes opportunities to involve the patient in the decision-making and his or her own management.

Langewitz *et al.* (1998) suggest specific interviewing skills:

- Help the patient clarify his/her concerns.
- Find relevant information.
- Offer a negotiation process.
- Invite patient participation in decision-making.
- Empathy in greeting behavior.
- Acknowledging initial complaints.
- Take up emotions instead of suppressing them.
- Clarify consultation reasons.
- Summarising patient's statement in doctor's own words.
- Summarising, acknowledging initial complaints, clarify purpose of the consultation.
- Explicit announcement of history-taking phase.
- Generally structuring the consultation.

- Shared evaluation of the consultation.
- Convey information as detailed as possible and as desired by the patient, ie results and preliminary diagnosis, aetiology, prognosis; communicate about treatment options, feasibility of treatment, future prospects.

Maguire & Pitceathly (2002) identify the following key tasks in communication with patients:

- Eliciting (a) the patient's main problems; (b) the patient's perceptions of these; and (c) the physical, emotional, and social impact of the patient's problems on the patient and family.
- Tailoring information to what the patient wants to know; checking his or her understanding.
- Eliciting the patient's reactions to the information given and his or her main concerns.
- Determining how much the patient wants to participate in decision-making (when treatment options are available).
- Discussing treatment options so that the patient understands the implications.
- Maximising the chance that the patient will follow agreed decisions about treatment and advice about changes in lifestyle.

Keller & Carroll (1994) quote Bird & Cohen-Cole (1991) who developed the idea of an interview having three functions: (a) gathering data to understand the patient; (b) development of rapport and responding to the patient's emotions; and (c) patient education and behavioural management.

Silverman *et al.* (2005), in the *Cambridge-Calgary guides*, describe five basic tasks that 'physicians and patients routinely attempt to accomplish in everyday clinical practice: initiating the session, gathering information, building the relationship, explanation and planning, and closing the session.' They state that this was first proposed by Riccardi and Kurz (1983). Cegala & Broz (2002) report that 'the Silverman *et al.* approach is structured entirely by interview stages and functions and is in our judgement one of the most comprehensive, useful frameworks available for instruction in provider communication skills.'

Silverman *et al.* (2005) take the view that 'building the relationship and structuring the interview are tasks that occur throughout the interview rather than sequentially. Both of these continuous tasks are essential for the five sequential tasks to be completed successfully.'

Building the relationship includes:

- Appropriate nonverbal behaviour; eye contact, facial expression, posture, position, movement, vocal cues;
- If reads, writes notes or uses computer, does so in a manner that does not interfere with dialogue or rapport;
- Demonstrates appropriate confidence;
- Develops rapport; accepts, is not judgemental; uses empathy; overtly acknowledges patient's views and feelings;
- Provides support, offers partnership;
- Deals sensitively with embarrassing and disturbing topics and physical pain;
- Involving the patient: shares thinking, explains rationale and, during physical examination, explains process.

Providing structure to the consultation includes:

- Making organisation overt; summarises at the end of a specific line of enquiry;
- Progresses from one section to another using signposting and transitional statements; includes rationale for next section;
- Attending to flow: structures interview in logical sequence;
- Attends to timing and keeping interview on task.

Opening the session

Lipkin (1996) mentions that preparing the environment is an important first step in the consultation process; making sure that there is a quiet, comfortable, and private place in which you can interview the patient. The next step is preparing oneself by eliminating distractions, having a means of focusing the mind, through meditation or constructive imaging, and letting intrusive thoughts pass.

Kalet *et al.* (2004) also recommend that preparation includes review of the patient's notes, and an assessment of your own personal issues (values, biases and assumptions) going into the encounter.

The consultation is then opened by greeting the patient, introducing oneself, and inviting the patient to make himself comfortable. It may be useful at this point to explain your role, and to say how much time is available for the consultation. You can then go on to establish the reason for the patient's visit, outline an agenda, and make a personal connection (Makoul, 2001).

Gathering information and questioning

This section of the interview focuses on 'question/answer framing, working from open to closed questions, reflecting questions, silence without interruption, facilitation, response to verbal and non-verbal cues, clarification, summarising, and the negotiation of plans' (RCP, 1997).

Maguire (2000) makes the point that the traditional directive style of interviewing – the doctor asking patients what their main complaints are and then asking rote questions about specific symptoms – has been shown to be relatively ineffective in promoting patient disclosure, and key problems may not be revealed.

Tate (2007) reports that:

> *doctors make hypotheses very early on in a consultation – usually in the first 30 seconds, sometimes even earlier. Once you have made a hypothesis, for example, 'this woman has toxic multinodular goitre,' all of your energies are channelled towards proving that hypothesis. There follows a rapid-fire series of clinical, closed questions directed towards that end, to the exclusion of a broader picture. You will gain so much more valuable information by consciously delaying your first hypothesis for, say, just one minute.*

Hargie & Dickson (2004) state that 'a question is only as good as the response it produces.' They quote a study (Sanchez, 2001) in which, during an average consultation time per patient of 2.1 minutes, doctors asked 27.3 questions. It is easy to slip into a pattern of asking several questions at once, or to ask another question before the patient has had time to answer the last. Or to be focusing so intently on the next question you want to ask that you find you haven't heard the patient's response at all.

So how should we be asking questions? Kalet *et al.* (2004) suggest starting with open-ended, non-focused questions, then inviting the patient to tell the story chronologically ('narrative thread'). Listening without interrupting allows the patient to state all of his or her concerns. Saying 'Tell me more,' 'What else?' and nodding all provide encouragement.

Simpson *et al.* (1991) state that 'the appropriate use of open ended questions, frequent summaries, clarification and negotiation are factors that positively affect the quality and quantity of information gathered; factors with a negative impact include inappropriate use of closed ended questions and premature advice or reassurance.' Cegala & Broz (2002) point out that it is the timing and placement of open questions rather than their frequency which appears to be important.

Stewart & Roter (1989) state that 'we analyse whether the doctor acknowledges or cuts off the patient's expression of ideas, expectations, feelings, or prompts. An acknowledgement is defined as a verbal indication that the physician has heard the patient.'

Maguire & Pitceathly (2002) suggest that in order to elicit patients' problems and concerns, the doctor should:

> *establish and maintain eye contact; ask for dates of key events and about patients' perceptions and feelings; clarify what patients are concerned about; respond to cues about problems and distress; avoid interrupting; summarise information, and enquire about the social and psychological impact of important illnesses or problems on the patient and family.*

Makoul (2001) describes several steps for eliciting information:

- Elicit patient's view of problem and/or progress (ideas, concerns).
- Explore physical/physiological factors (signs, symptoms).
- Explore psychosocial/emotional factors (living situation, family relations, stress).

- Discuss antecedent treatments (self-care, last visit, other care).
- Discuss how health problems affect the patient's life.
- Discuss lifestyle issues/prevention strategies (health risks).
- Check/clarify information.

Maguire *et al.* (1996a) found that three behaviours promote patient disclosure of key concerns: open directive questions, questions with a psychological focus and clarification of psychological aspects. In contrast, they found that behaviours which inhibit disclosure included the use of questions with a physical focus, utterances clarifying physical aspects and the giving of advice prematurely.

Levenstein *et al.* (1989) defined 'all statements not acknowledged by the physician as cut-offs: the physician blocks the patient's further expression of ideas, expectations, or feelings by changing the subject, using closed-ended or rhetorical questions, or not acknowledging a prompt.' Lang *et al.* (2002) state that 'without special efforts the patient's perspective on illness (PPI) surfaces spontaneously in only about one fourth of medical interviews.' Interestingly, they found that doctors felt less helpful to patients who revealed their ideas and concerns during the interview.

Hargie & Dickson (2004) quote West (1983), who found that only 9% of questions were initiated by patients, and Wynn (1996), who found that medical students quickly learned to handle patient-initiated questions by asking unrelated doctor-initiated ones which maintained control of the consultation.

Keller & Carroll (1994) state that patients have questions that they do not always ask, and that doctors should assume that they want to know:

1. What has happened to me?
2. Why has it happened to me?
3. What is going to happen to me, in the short term, in the long-term?

They also advise doctors to answer questions about their actions, and to assume that patients want to know:

1.   What are you doing to me (examination, tests)?
2.   Why are you doing this rather than something else?
3.   Will it hurt me or harm me, for how long and how much?
4.   When and how will you know what these tests mean?
5.   When and how will I know what these tests mean?

Shilling *et al.* (2003) found that 'patient satisfaction was influenced by the simple act of asking if they have any questions during the consultation and by trying to ensure that the patient does not leave with unanswered questions.'

Hargie & Dickson (2004) report that the overwhelming focus of practitioner-patient interaction is task-centred, concerns the discussion of physical symptoms and tends to ignore the emotional aspects of the patient's well-being (Gilmore & Hargie, 2000), and that the 'dearth of questions relating to the affective domain is the main reason for the poor rate of detection of psychosocial problems in patients' (Dickson *et al.*, 1997).

Stewart *et al.* (1995) recommend that 'an interviewing style that seeks to elicit signs and symptoms of physical illness but also demonstrates a genuine interest in the patient as a person early in the interview, and seeks to cover physical and psychological aspects, is much more effective in promoting honest disclosure' (Maguire, 2000).

Platt *et al.* (2001) outline five areas of concern in getting to know the patient as a person:

1.   Who is this patient? What constitutes that person's life? What are the patient's interests, work, important relationships, major concerns?
2.   What does this patient want from the physician? What are their values and fears? What do they hope to accomplish here today or in the long run?
3.   How does this patient experience this illness? Specifically, what has it done to him functionally; how has it affected relationships; and what symbolic meaning does it hold for him?
4.   What are the patient's ideas about the illness? What is their understanding and perception of the disorder and its cause? What would seem to be reasonable treatment for it?

5.   What are the patient's main feelings about the illness, with special attention to the five common responses: fear, distrust, anger, sadness, and ambivalence?

Coulter *et al.* (1999) suggest that patients frequently would like the answers to these questions:

- Is it essential to have treatment for this problem?
- Will the treatment(s) relieve the symptoms?
- How long will it take to recover?
- What are the possible side effects?
- What effect will the treatment(s) have on my feelings and emotions?
- What effect will the treatment(s) have on my sex life?
- What do my carers need to know?
- What can I do to speed recovery?
- What are the options for rehabilitation?
- How can I prevent recurrence or future illness?
- Where can I get more information about the problem or treatments?

Haidet & Paterniti (2003) suggest that practitioners adopt a 'narrative-based medicine' approach to the medical interview by:

- Simultaneously attending to two narratives: one from the biomedical perspective and one from the patient's perspective;
- Starting with open-ended questions and gradually increasing the focus, or 'close-endedness' of questions;
- Using other conversational devices such as orientation statements, paraphrasing statements, reflections, and directives.

They conclude that building a history in this way and allowing the patient to express his or her own perspectives means that a shared understanding can be reached.

Explanation and planning

It is important to explain to the patient in easily understandable language what you are going to do, and the reasons for doing it, during a physical examination or procedure, or if further investigations are needed.

In terms of diagnosis, Keller & Carroll (1994) point out that 'most patients make a self-diagnosis... If your diagnosis and the patient's differ, the patient will act based upon his or her own diagnosis. Consequently, it is imperative that you understand and discuss the patient's diagnosis.' Beckman *et al.* (1989) quote Kleinman *et al.* (1978) who suggested several useful questions to determine the impact of a problem on a patient's social and emotional context:

- What do you think caused your problems?
- Why do you think it started when it did?
- How severe is your sickness?
- What are the most important results you hope to achieve?
- What do you fear most about your sickness?

Patients have a need for information about diagnosis, prognosis, condition or treatment to be delivered in ways that they can understand (Hargie & Dickson, 2004). Tate (2007) points out that:

> *the MRCGP Consulting Skills module (November 2000) has shown achieving shared understanding to be the rarest of all observed behaviours, with less than 5% of doctors demonstrating it in three out of five selected consultations. Strategically positioned computer screens should be visible to the patient and a focus for sharing information. A study of MRCGP candidates in 2000 demonstrated that this actually occurs in less than 10% of surgeries.*

Explanation needs to proceed at a rate that the patient is comfortable with, and is able to process. Fear and anxiety are frequent inhibitors of both understanding and recall. Poor concordance may be related to patients forgetting important details of treatment or medication. It is important that an agreement can be reached about what doctor and patient feel the problem is. If there is agreement on diagnosis and management, then the patient is more likely to follow the treatment plan.

The Royal College of Physicians' report (1997) states that:

> *Doctors may be unaware of the need to structure their explanations (for example, warning the patient what is going to be discussed,*

*summarising at the end, allowing the patient time to ask questions).
They may fail to couch explanations in simple, clear language or
to pace the rate at which information and explanations are given.
Clear and simple language is important; failure to use it can
become a major source of dissatisfaction. Doctors may not sense
what a patient is ready to receive/understand, either emotionally
or intellectually. Patients need to feel that the doctor is listening
to them and is prepared to discuss or answer their questions.*

Silverman *et al.*. (2005) state that the aims with explanation are to
give comprehensive and appropriate information; to assess each
individual patient's information needs; to neither restrict nor
overload. To this end they suggest the doctor:

- Chunks and checks; gives information in assimilable chunks;
  checks for understanding; uses patient's response as a guide
  to how to proceed;
- Assesses patient's starting point; asks for patient's
  prior knowledge; discovers extent of patient's wish for
  information;
- Asks patient what other information would be helpful;
- Gives explanation at appropriate times, not prematurely;
- Uses repetition and summarising: encourages patients to
  contribute;
- Negotiates a mutually acceptable plan; checks patient's
  concerns have been addressed.

Maguire & Pitceathly (2002) present a checklist for giving
information:

- Check what patients consider might be wrong;
- Ask patients what information they would like;
- Present information by category – for example, 'you said you
  would like to know the nature of your illness.'
- Check that the patient has understood.
- Discuss treatment options and check if patients want to be
  involved in decisions. Determine the patient's perspective
  before discussing lifestyle changes – for example, giving up
  smoking.
- Be supportive and show that you have some sense of how
  the patient is feeling ('the experiences you describe during
  your mother's illness sound devastating.')

- Feed back to patients your intuitions about how they are feeling ('you say you are coping well, but I get the impression you are struggling with this treatment.')

Dowell *et al.* (2002) state that a sensitive, structured exploration of patients' beliefs can explain medication use and expose barriers to change, noting that it is especially important for patients and doctors to understand how they are each evaluating the treatment's effects. They suggest a model to assist concordant prescribing which explores patients' feelings about their diagnosis and treatment:

- 'Tell me about when your diagnosis was made?'
- 'What does this diagnosis mean to you?'
- 'How do you feel about your treatment?'
- 'How do you judge if it is working?'
- 'How do you use your treatment?'

Coulter *et al.* (1999) found that most patients 'indicated a preference for information that is balanced and includes a careful and honest assessment of the pros and cons of treatment. If outcome probabilities are unknown because relevant research has not been carried out, it is best to be frank about this rather than provide reassurance that may turn out to be false.' Roter (1989) noted that 'physician expressions of uncertainty to patients are consistent with an increasingly accepted model of care that values information exchange and shared decision-making over physician certainty and control.' Gordon *et al.* (2000) quote Hewson *et al.* (1996) who described steps for 'strategic medical management' of uncertain and complex medical problems, including acknowledging and discussing uncertainty.

As Elwyn *et al.* (2001) point out, choices legitimately exist in most clinical situations. Few interventions are risk free (Thornton, 2003). Kennedy (2003) states that the communication of risk in numerical terms is by no means always appropriate or meaningful for patients. Edwards (2003) states that while experts may think of risk as derived from scientific research, patients want to know whether or how they will be affected. The goal is to inform people, enabling them to make their own choices, regardless of whether this reduces risk. Then, communication of risk occurs within the context of shared decision-making (Godolphin, 2003).

Closing the session

At the end of the session, it is a good idea to briefly summarise the plan, and ask if the patient has any questions or other issues to discuss. Kalet states that, having arrived at a mutually acceptable solution, it is sensible to check the patient's willingness and ability to follow the plan. Then, clarify what to do in the interim, establish a safety net, schedule the next encounter and say goodbye (Lipkin, 1996).

Chapter 5
How to improve communication

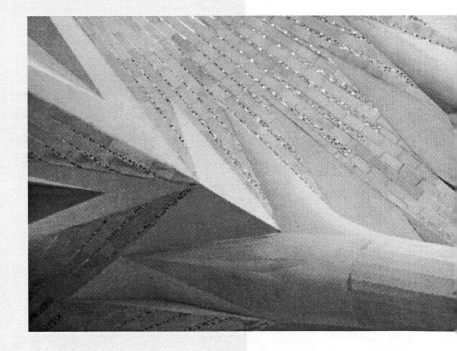

How to improve communication

The patient-centred approach: a model for clinical interviewing

The term 'patient-centred medicine' was introduced by Balint *et al.* (1970) who contrasted it with 'illness-centred medicine.' The illness centred consultation has been described by other writers as doctor-centred or disease-centred (Levenstein, 1989).

Byrne and Long (1976) reported that:

> *the patient-centred method is characterised by use of the patient's knowledge and experience; the doctor uses silence, listening and reflecting; clarifying and interpreting. This method stems from a belief in the ability of the patient to make decisions and to be involved in his own treatment.*

The doctor-centred method uses the doctor's skill and special knowledge; gathering information, analysing and probing.

Stewart & Roter (1989) state that the patient-centred method aims not just at diagnosis of disease but also at understanding the meaning of the illness for the patient. It requires an ability to listen attentively, to be empathic and to pick up on and respond to patients' emotional cues. The authors also draw attention to the fact that:

> *The patient-centred method requires a radical change in the very person of the physician, in the definition of the medical task, and in the basic epistemology of medicine. Medical education must encourage reflection, personal development, and the growth of self-knowledge. It must also teach communication skills that reveal the patient's world to the physician, and analytic skills that can encompass a complex web of relationships rather than single causal chains.*

This suggests that doctors need to develop a range of capacities which are not strictly communication skills, but are more closely related to values and attitudes to the therapeutic relationship. Roter (2000) states that: 'incorporation of the patient's perspective into a relationship-centred medical paradigm has been suggested as appropriate for the 21st Century.' This chapter will explore this further.

The benefits of improved communication

Levenstein *et al.* (1989) write that 'most patients have their own thoughts about what is wrong with them, what might be causing it, and what might be its implications.' Patients should be involved in their own care, and have a sense of control over their own treatment (Stewart & Roter, 1989). Tate (2007) quotes Stimpson & Webb (1975) who point out that although 'in the consultation the doctor makes the treatment decisions; after the consultation, decision making lies with the patient.' The doctor must therefore investigate the patient's ideas, concerns and expectations as part of the management process (Pendleton *et al.*, 1984 in Thistlethwaite & Jordan, 1999).

Little *et al.* (2001a) found that 'patients in primary care strongly want a patient-centred approach, with communication, partnership, and health promotion.' Batenburg *et al.* (1999) report that several studies have affirmed that patient-centred attitudes are most apparent among psychiatrists, followed by general practitioners, while doctor-centred attitudes are prominent among surgeons. Roter *et al.* (2002) carried out a meta-analysis of twenty-six communication studies, and found that women doctors are more likely to engage patients as active partners in decision making, to elicit patient preferences, and to be sensitive to their psychosocial and emotional concerns.

However, few studies have investigated the effect of patient characteristics on preferences for different styles of communication in doctors. Graugaard & Finset (2000) conducted an interesting study in which the emotional state of 20 students with low trait anxiety was compared with that of 21 students with high trait anxiety following a consultation which was either patient-centred or doctor-centred. They found that:

> *students with low trait anxiety were significantly more satisfied with a patient-centred than a doctor-centred communication style, whereas among the students with high trait anxiety, no significant difference was found. The trend for the latter tended more toward*

> *satisfaction with a doctor-centred communication style. Those students with a high level of trait anxiety who experienced a patient-centred intervention reacted emotionally most negatively immediately after the consultation.*

Stewart (1995) reported that doctors provide most patients with partially patient-centred care, and Stewart (2001) found that on a patient-centred rating scale of 0-100, the average was 50.7. This is low, considering that patient-centred consulting has been shown to increase patient satisfaction (Kinnersley *et al.*, 1999), enhance outcomes of care including patient adherence to treatment recommendations, improve biological outcomes in chronic disease (Kaplan *et al.*, 1989; Levinson & Lurie, 2004); and increase the efficiency of care by reducing diagnostic tests and referrals (Stewart *et al.*, 2000).

Empathy

Batenburg *et al.* (1999) write that in general practice, many problems cannot be diagnosed neatly, and many contain psychological and social elements. Stewart *et al.* (2000) quote a number of studies which show that 'psychosocial and psychiatric problems are common in general medical practice, but these diagnoses are missed in up to 50% of cases (Schulberg & Burns, 1988; Freeling *et al.*, 1985).' Even as far back as 1957, Balint recognised that 'at least one-quarter to one-third of the work of the general practitioner consists of psychotherapy pure and simple. Present medical training does not properly equip the practitioner for at least a quarter of the work he has to do.'

In other words, medicine was never solely a question of diagnosis and management of illness. Also of vital importance was the relationship with the patient, the offering of a therapeutic space in which patients could express their concerns and receive support and advice.

In 1979, Poole & Sanson-Fisher wrote of 'a vast body of research data which demonstrates that there are a number of core facilitative qualities, eg accurate empathy, genuineness and non-possessive warmth, which are important aspects of the interviewing and therapeutic processes.' According to Coulehan *et al.* (2001):

numerous investigators have demonstrated the importance of empathy in the medical encounter. Empathy allows the patient to feel understood, respected and validated. This promotes diagnostic accuracy, therapeutic adherence, and patient satisfaction, while remaining time-efficient. Empathy also enhances physician satisfaction.

So what is empathy? According to Disiker & Michielutte (1981) it is 'the ability to understand what another person is experiencing and to communicate that understanding to the person.' They suggest that empathy is a multidimensional construct that includes more than the ability to communicate effectively. It is questionable, however, to what degree we are ever going to able to understand someone else's experience if it is widely divergent from our own. To say 'I understand how you must feel' can lead patients to take offence or to mistrust your motives. If you have never experienced chronic pain, or the loss of a loved one, or childhood abuse, then when you say you understand, many patients will sense the lack of genuineness in your statement.

Bub (2006) states emphatically: 'Never ever say, "I understand how you feel." You don't and this expression is highly alienating.'

So what could be used instead? Some alternatives could be:

- 'That sounds very upsetting... How have you managed?'
- 'That must have been a very difficult time... How did you cope with all of that?'
- 'What an awful situation, were you frightened?'

The important thing is to let the patient know that you are trying to understand, and that you are giving them time and space to express what their feelings, if they are able. Their emotional position is validated by the fact that you are acknowledging how they might have felt, even though you don't know:

- 'I can't even begin to imagine how that must have felt for you.'
- 'That must have been totally devastating...' and then leave silence.

Matthews *et al.* (1993) states that:

> *as we develop a fuller understanding, we are then in a position to let the patient know that we understand. This may take various forms: a simple empathic statement ('You've really been through a lot'); legitimation ('I can see why you would have found that difficult'); self-disclosure ('I went through a situation like that once; I felt the same way'); a rephrasing or summarization of the patient's situation ('Let me make sure I understand what you've been telling me'); or a comment about one's own immediate responses to the patient's story ('It makes me sad to hear that') (Cohen-Cole, 1991).*

Beach *et al.* (2004) conducted some interesting research into the effects of physician self-disclosure, which was defined as 'a statement describing the physician's personal experience that has medical and/or emotional relevance for the patient.' Generally, 71% of physicians self-disclose, regardless of speciality. In Beach *et al.*'s study, self-disclosure occurred in 17% of primary care visits and 14% of surgical visits. Self-disclosure was significantly associated with higher patient satisfaction ratings for surgical visits and lower patient satisfaction ratings for primary care visits.

In other words, in some situations it can be helpful to talk about your own personal experiences. For example in discussing smoking with a patient:

Patient: 'I have stopped for a week, I felt so bad with the flu I just didn't want to smoke.'

Doctor: 'That's fantastic, well done. That's a great achievement. Do you want to keep off it?'

Patient: 'Yeah, I reckon I've gone through the worst already.'

Doctor: 'You probably have. Quitting smoking... it's the hardest thing you ever do. But it is doable. I smoked for twenty-five years and I finally did it. But we're addicts, we make all sorts of excuses, don't we? We're really good at finding reasons not to stop...'

Your experience may serve as encouragement to others:

> Doctor: 'Would you agree to see someone to talk about all this stuff? It won't go away.'
>
> Patient: 'I don't want people to think I'm a nutter or anything like that, they think you are if you say you're seeing a counsellor.'
>
> Doctor: 'I think therapy is the most important thing you ever do in your life.'
>
> Patient: 'Do you do it?'
>
> Doctor: 'Yes, of course. My therapist is a really nice woman. And once you've been going a while, it does get easier to tell people about it.'

Poole & Sanson-Fisher (1979) quote Truax and Carkhuff (1967) who define accurate empathy as 'the ability to be sensitive to another's current feelings and the verbal facility to communicate this understanding in a language attuned to the patient's present feelings.' Keller & Carroll (1994) note that empathy conveys an impression that the physician is 'present' and 'with' the patient. They quote Spiro *et al.* (1993) who state that 'empathy can be seen as an active concern for and curiosity about the emotions, values, and experiences of another.'

In order to be present, the doctor must be focused on the patient, and emotionally available. Matthews *et al.* (1993) make the point that:

> *as the patient begins to relate his story, it is necessary to silence our own internal talk – that part of consciousness that is already forming the next comment, question, or criticism, even as the patient is still speaking, distracting our attention away from his experience and from our own spontaneous responses. The diagnostic reasoning process, too, is a kind of internal talk that can interfere with our ability to listen; it can safely be deferred for a few moments until the patient's story is completed.*

This means being aware not just of our own agenda – our need to make an assessment, an accurate diagnosis and a working plan for management of the problem – but also of our own feelings as the interview progresses. Junior doctors, for example, are expected to assess and manage a wide range of disorders which they may or may not feel comfortable with. They may feel under-confident, lacking in technical ability or theoretical knowledge, or personally inadequate to the task. The patient may trigger feelings in them which are hard to acknowledge or deal with. The interview may be punctuated by feelings of losing the thread, not being sure where to go next, or of panic. In other words, the anxieties of the doctor can dominate the interview. The doctor's thoughts of what they should be doing, worries about what they may have forgotten, or intermittent anxiety about time pressure, may interrupt their flow of being in the present and prevent them from being emotionally available to the patient.

Haidet & Paterniti (2003) talk of 'mindful practice' as the ability of the physician to observe not only the patient during the medical interview, but himself as well. Zoppi & Epstein (2002) write about mindful 'being-in-relation' as a way of viewing the patient-doctor relationship. They state that mindful physicians can easily be identified by patients and colleagues – they are present, attentive, curious and unhindered by preconceptions.

This concern on the part of the doctor is important to the patient. It communicates something like: 'Let's put our heads together to think about the problems. We're looking at this together. We both want to find a solution.' And, perhaps more importantly, that 'it matters to me what's happening to you.' You are allies with a common bond, grappling with the problem, or illness, or issue, trying to find the best way to deal with it and even overcome it.

Skelton *et al.* (2002) suggest the pattern is:

> 'Patient: I suffer.
> Doctor: I think.
>
> We will act.
>
> The patient brings the problem, the doctor brings rational expertise to bear on it, and offers partnership in action.'

In Chapter 3 the importance of nonverbal communication was noted. Zoppi & Epstein (2002) state that 'inflections, gestures and eye contact are rarely included in communication skills training.' It is therefore not uncommon for an individual doctor not to be aware of his or her own nonverbal messages and behaviour. Coulehan *et al.* (2001) stress that active listening requires 'nonverbal and paralanguage skills, such as appropriate position and posture; good eye contact; mirroring of facial expression; and facilitative responses, such as nodding and minimal expressions.'

It is interesting to observe that medical students and junior doctors frequently do not show much facial expression as they listen to a patient's story. Even when events are reported that were intensely upsetting for the patient, they may not show sympathetic facial expressions. While feeling sympathy or concern, they may not be actually communicating this. Roter & Hall (2006) state that 'there is research suggesting that primary care doctors do poorly at recognizing patients' emotional distress, perhaps because they fail to fully attend to emotional cues.'

DiMatteo & Taranta (1979) examined the nonverbal communication skills of doctors as predictors of their ability to establish rapport with their patients. In exploring the role of nonverbal sensitivity and expressiveness (decoding and encoding skill), they found that 'the socioemotional dimension of the physician-patient relationship depends, to a moderate degree at least, on the physician's ability to understand the patient's nonverbal cues of affect and on the physician's ability intentionally to communicate affect through nonverbal channels.' They made the point that the literature at the time showed that measures of intellectual ability and performance were poor predictors of physicians' interpersonal effectiveness.

Coulehan *et al.* (2001) define empathy as 'the ability to understand the patient's situation, perspective, and feelings and to communicate that understanding to the patient.' They suggest that this is done by asking questions to understand the patient's thoughts and feelings, and gaining feedback by checking with the patient what has been understood of their situation, for example using statements such as 'Let me see if I have this right.'

It makes sense to find out what the patient thinks is wrong, or their opinion of past diagnoses, for instance.

- 'What do you think? What's your view?'
- 'What diagnosis have you been given? Do you agree? Would something else suit your symptoms better? What would your diagnosis be?'

Many patients have read up on their condition and other related conditions on the Internet, and have their own views on diagnosis and management. The diagnosis that a patient has been given is not necessarily right. It is best not to assume that the old diagnosis is correct, rather to find out yourself what the story has been, and, if necessary, to go back to the beginning so that your view is unconstrained by past definitions which may have been limiting. If new information comes to light, it can be a great relief to a patient to be given a more accurate diagnosis.

Rapport

Matthews *et al.* (1993) suggest that the most basic element of connection is rapport, which depends on mutual respect and interest between clinician and patient. Their view is that 'recognition and explicit acknowledgment of emotional content in the patient's story is particularly important in establishing rapport.' If you are interested in how a person feels about what has happened to them, then they will sense that you care, not just about their illness or problem, but about them as an individual as well. Stewart (2005) quotes Tarlow (1996) who defines caring as 'a process encompassing eight concepts: time, being there, talking, sensitivity, acting in the best interest of the other, feeling, doing and reciprocity.'

Hall *et al.* (1995) write that 'rapport is characterised by mutual attentiveness or involvement, and high levels of positivity or warmth.' Levinson *et al.* (2000) quote Suchman *et al.* (1997) who suggested that 'physicians often "terminate" the empathic opportunity by changing the topic from the patient's emotional concerns to a salient biomedical issue that seems to be a more comfortable topic for physicians.' They found that doctors miss opportunities presented by patients through failure to adequately acknowledge patients' feelings, inappropriate humour, terminating the topic, and denial of patient emotion.

Maguire & Pitceathly (2002) state that doctors respond to emotional cues with strategies that block further disclosure:

- Offering advice and reassurance before the main problems have been identified.
- Explaining away distress as normal.
- Attending to physical aspects only.
- Switching the topic.
- 'Jollying' patients along.

Without listening to the patient's story, the doctor cannot form an accurate assessment of what the patient feels about his illness. It is important to gain some idea of how the patient responds to stress, how they deal with emotions such as anger, fear and sadness, and what ego strengths they have at their disposal, in addition to their social network of support. To show interest in these areas helps the doctor to determine the impact that illness may have. Many patients have their own ideas of what has contributed to or caused their illness, and will want to tell the doctor. The doctor needs to be aware of these ideas in order to negotiate a mutual understanding which accommodates both views. If the doctor does not listen, ask or respond to the patient's thoughts and feelings, they are invalidating the patient's perspective.

Smith & Hoppe (1991) state that:

> *according to the biopsychosocial model every patient has a story that demonstrates the interaction among the biologic, psychologic, and social components of his or her life. Gestalt theory posits that people are continuously developing a story that portrays what is most important in their lives. The patient's story emerges in a meaningful, integrated, and complete way. The physician's task is to elicit and understand this story, for it provides an introduction to who the person is and why he or she is seeing the physician. The story also provides clues to diagnostic and therapeutic issues relevant to the patient's problem.*

Charon (2001) states that 'as in psychoanalysis, in all of medical practice the narrating of the patient's story is a therapeutically central act, because to find the words to contain the disorder and its attendant worries gives shape to and control over the chaos of illness.' Narrative medicine is proposed as a model for humane and effective medical practice. Bury (2001) writes that 'the starting point for much of the current interest in illness narratives has been

103

the perceived need (Kleinman, 1988) to "witness" the suffering of those with serious, and especially disabling chronic disorders.'

Mercer & Howie (2006) state that patients consistently rank empathy and humanness as a key attribute of a 'good doctor.' Coulter (2002b), in a systematic review of the literature on patients' priorities for general practice care, found that the most highly rated aspect of care was 'humaneness.' This was followed by 'competence/accuracy,' 'patients' involvement in decisions,' and 'time for care.' Levinson *et al.* (2000) confirms that outcomes of care are optimal when physicians address patients' emotional and personal concerns in addition to their biomedical problems.

Relationship

Stewart (2004) posits four central questions regarding the patient-clinician relationship: 'What is it? What aspects do patients expect and value? What can clinicians do or not do that will support the development of a positive and therapeutic relationship? What are the benefits of a positive relationship?'

Zoppi & Epstein (2002) quote Candib (1995) who states that 'an interaction is characterised by an observable exchange of behaviours, whereas a relationship is characterised by more subjective qualities, such as caring, concern, respect and compassion.' They also make the point that 'the received effect of a relationship on a patient is only loosely correlated with observational data about communication.' In other words, it may be possible to observe specific communication skills or behaviours which a doctor demonstrates in a consultation with a patient, but the relationship that exists between them is not measured simply by the presence or absence of these skills. The quality of the relationship as perceived by the patient is something that is rarely measured or investigated. According to Zoppi & Epstein (2002), 'it is likely that there are frequent discrepancies between patients' and physicians' sense of being connected, in tune with each other, congruent emotionally, and moving toward the same goals.' They use the term intersubjectivity to describe this connection.

So what is the doctor-patient relationship? Aspects highlighted as important – by doctors at least – are respect, dignity and trust. Branch (2006) states that 'to show respect is to show esteem, regard or honour to another person. To be respectful is also to be humble. Respect is a core value of medical professionalism.' Beach *et al.* (2005) report that 'although involving patients in decisions is an important part of respecting patient autonomy, it is also important to respect patients more broadly by treating them with dignity.'

The Royal College of Physicians Report (2005) states that doctors aim to restore and strengthen both well-being and a patient's dignity:

> *Dignity emphasises ... the intrinsic moral worth of a human being and also the freedom and capacity – physical and mental – of the individual to live a life that they desire. Behaviours that strengthen trust include courtesy, kindness, understanding, humility, honesty, and confidentiality. These behaviours create an environment of safety around the patient.*

In terms of the aspects that patients value, Kirsner (2009) tells how he asked a patient which member of the medical team the patient would most like as his personal doctor. The patient chose the medical student because: 'he visited me every evening; asked about my family, what I did for a living, about things that might be bothering me. He was the only one who talked to me, explained everything, and encouraged me. He's a real doctor.'

Barnett (2001) quotes Miller and Rollnick, who state that: 'the client must feel that the clinician can be trusted, genuinely cares, and is interested in trying to help.' Hargie & Dickson (2004) noted that:

> *one in-depth study of listening dyads found that what speakers most wanted was for the listener to understand what they were saying, and to care about and empathise with them – their recommendation was to 'listen with your heart' (Halone & Pecchioni, 2001). This type of listening is common between close friends and spouses. It is at the core of formal helping situations, and hence has also been termed therapeutic listening (Wolvin & Coakley, 1996).*

Byrne & Long (1976) were of the view that 'two human beings go through a series of manoeuvres to discover whether or not the other party is prepared to listen to what they really want to say. Shooting down at any stage usually indicates that there is not a relationship of confidence and nothing of moment will be said.'

It is very important to realise that if patients are stopped short when attempting to say something which is difficult, upsetting or important for them, then they probably will not keep trying. As Bub (2006) states, healing emerges from healing relationships: 'patients intuit your willingness to listen and will share private information. It will always be significant, and patients will rarely abuse your time. Almost invariably, this results in improvement in medical care.'

Matthews *et al.* (1993) quote Rogers (1961):

> *beyond feeling understood, patients may often need to feel accepted. After personal feelings come to light, they may feel surprised, embarrassed, and vulnerable to judgment, mockery, or rejection on the part of the listener. Having encouraged patients to explore these deeper levels of meaning, it becomes our responsibility to show them compassion and unconditional acceptance.*

Tomm (1988) defines therapeutic conversations as those which are organised by the desire to relieve mental pain and suffering and to produce healing: 'some patterns of conversing are much more conducive to being therapeutic than others – for example, asking questions stimulates clients to think through their problems on their own.'

Neighbour (2005) describes how, watching someone who is good at consulting, 'you would be aware of a sense of flow, of depth beneath the surface exchanges, of more complex things happening than the purely clinical agenda would suggest. You might notice unexpected flashes of insight in either doctor or patient, or upsurges of emotion – sadness, fear, anger – leading the consultation towards greater truthfulness.'

Bub (2006) explains that 'for communication to heal it needs to be authentic, ie it needs to emerge from the authentic self. This form of communication is by definition highly personal since how you listen and what you say emerges from you, and not from lifeless parroting of scripted information.'

However, many authors describe the problems that doctors face in defining a professional self. Salinsky & Sackin (2000) take the view that a good doctor-patient relationship needs the involvement of the personal self:

> *We may come to believe that it is possible and desirable to develop a 'professional self' who handles all our business activities and is unaffected by human emotions. Meanwhile the 'personal self' inhabits a different space inside us and is never affected by the emotions of our patients. It is through our personal self that we make contact with the patient as one human being with another. If we try to shut the personal self away when we see our patients they are deprived of the empathy and warmth that enables them to feel that they have been truly heard and that they are cared for.*

Bub (2006) states that:

> *emotions are essential for empathy, compassion, communication, and healing. The more comfortable a physician is with her own emotions, the more she is able to tolerate and even welcome the emotions of others. Do not suppress the emotions of others with premature reassurance or words of comfort. To the extent that you are comfortable with your emotions, you will feel comfortable being with the emotions of others and be able to accept them without yours getting in the way.*

Groopman (2008) quotes Peabody (1925): 'The secret of the care of the patient is in caring for the patient,' and adds that 'if we feel our emotions deeply, we risk recoiling or breaking down. If we erase our emotions, we fail to care for the patient.' A balance must be found, we must be willing to feel at least some of the patient's suffering and distress, otherwise we cannot provide support for what truly concerns him. We must be able to listen even if that is painful for us, and to encourage patients who may find it difficult to articulate their feelings. Frankel & Beckman (1989) point out that 'often the physician is perceived as the only person available to listen to and comfort distressed patients of all ages.'

Cox (1989) writes that 'with patients who tend to show emotion freely, the doctor only needs to be attentive, but with those who are more inhibited, the physician needs to question directly about feelings and to be more actively responsive when they are expressed.'

Salinsky & Sackin (2000) conclude that a mixture of objectivity and subjectivity seems to be necessary for good personal doctoring:

> *Balint (1987) described the way in which we as clinicians allow ourselves to approach closely, and identify with, a patient's feelings, to experience empathically something of their emotional state – and then step back again. By stepping back a little we can then examine the feelings we have experienced and consider what they mean. In this way we can also avoid being totally immersed in the patient's feelings and drowning before we can rescue them.*

The benefits of a positive relationship have been investigated in various studies. Frankel & Beckman (1989) report that 'patients were more satisfied if the doctor was warm (Francis *et al.*, 1969), empathic (Wasserman *et al.*, 1984), and allowed the patient to share opinions during the interview (Stewart, 1984).' MacDonald (2004) reports that 'the extent to which a doctor displays warmth, genuineness and unconditional regard for his patients also determines an effective therapeutic relationship (Rogers, 1951; Novak, 1987; Dixon *et al.*, 1999).' Roter *et al.* (2002) make the point that 'partnership building occurs when a physician actively facilitates patient participation in the medical visit or attempts to equalize status by assuming a less dominating stance within the relationship.' This may then allow the patient to be more open in expressing his or her feelings.

MacDonald (2004) reports the systematic review conducted by Di Blasi *et al.* (2000) which investigated the therapeutic effect of the doctor-patient relationship. 'It included eleven medical, psychological and sociological electronic databases, and reported the consistent finding that physicians who adopt a warm, friendly and reassuring manner are more effective in therapeutic terms than those who keep consultations formal and do not offer reassurance.'

Kaptchuk (2002) quotes studies which indicate that 'the patient-practitioner encounter is a potent factor in health outcomes and that for many non-life-threatening illnesses, clear diagnosis, assurance of recovery, opportunity for dialogue, and physician-patient agreement about the nature of the problem hasten recovery or relief.'

Emotional intelligence

An article in *The Times* entitled – perhaps not entirely helpfully – 'Why some doctors are rubbish' (January 23, 2007) quoted a study mentioned in the Health Service Journal assessing doctors whose performance had raised concerns to the degree that they had been referred to the National Clinical Assessment Service. The study allegedly reported that 'communication problems were frequent among this group of doctors. They may also be seen as emotionally volatile, narcissistic or arrogant. They can be extremely difficult to please and have poor self-awareness. They may be intellectually intelligent, but not emotionally.'

So what is emotional intelligence? McMullen (2002) writes that:

> *in 1983, Howard Gardner from the Harvard School of Education proposed that a single entity called intelligence does not exist. He put forward an idea of multiple intelligences: musical/rhythmic; visual/spatial; bodily/kinaesthetic; verbal/linguistic; logical/ mathematical; interpersonal; intrapersonal. Others have suggested different kinds of intelligences: cognitive (IQ), emotional (EQ), and spiritual (SQ).*

Traditionally, IQ was seen as an indicator of thinking abilities, and was measured by IQ tests such as the Wechsler Adult Intelligence Scale which placed an individual's performance on the normal distribution curve, the average IQ being 100. The currently used test, the WAIS-IV, (2008) scores verbal comprehension, perceptual reasoning, working memory and processing speed. Wechsler (1939) defined intelligence as 'The aggregate or global capacity of a person to act purposefully, to think rationally, and to deal effectively with his environment.'

Salovey & Mayer (1990) defined emotional intelligence (EI) as 'the ability to monitor one's own and others' feelings and emotions, to discriminate among them and to use this information to guide one's thinking and actions.' It focuses on how people appraise and communicate emotion, and how they use that emotion in solving problems and regulating behaviour. Their view was that:

> *when people approach life tasks with emotional intelligence, they should be at an advantage for solving problems adaptively. Having*

109

framed a problem, individuals with such skills may be more creative and flexible in arriving at possible alternatives to problems. They are also more apt to integrate emotional considerations when choosing among alternatives. Such an approach will lead to behaviour that is considerate and respectful of the internal experience of themselves and others.

The concept of EI was popularised by Goleman (1998) who defined an 'emotional competence' as a 'learned capability based on emotional intelligence that results in outstanding performance at work.' Boyatzis, Goleman & Rhee (1999) state that 'emotional intelligence is observed when a person demonstrates the competencies that constitute self-awareness, self-management, social awareness, and social skills at appropriate times and ways in sufficient frequency to be effective in the situation.'

However, there are two main reasons why we need to be cautious about embracing the idea of emotional intelligence *per se*. The first is that data are not available to confirm its value. Landy (2005) states:

It appears that emotional intelligence, as a concept related to occupational success, exists outside the typical scientific domain. Much of the data necessary for demonstrating the unique association between EI and work-related behaviour appears to reside in proprietary databases, preventing rigorous tests of the measurement devices or of their unique predictive value. For those reasons, any claims for the value of EI in the work setting cannot be made under the scientific mantle.

Secondly, various researchers have argued that the definition of emotional intelligence has become too varied or all-encompassing to be useful. For example, Locke (2005) argues that 'the concept of emotional intelligence (EI) is invalid both because it is not a form of intelligence and because it is defined so broadly and inclusively that it has no intelligible meaning... It is simply arbitrary to attach the word "intelligence" to assorted habits or skills, as Howard Gardner and EI advocates do, on the alleged grounds that there are multiple types of intelligences.'

Locke (2005) states that 'there is no common or integrating element in a concept that includes: introspection about emotions, emotional expression, non-verbal communication with others, empathy, self-regulation, planning, creative thinking and the direction of attention.'

Landy (2005) has claimed that 'the few incremental validity studies conducted on EI have demonstrated that it adds little or nothing to the explanation or prediction of some common outcomes (most notably academic and work success) (Van Rooy & Viswesvaran, 2004; Barchard, 2003; Brackett & Mayer, 2003).'

Finally, Locke (2005) makes the following conclusion about emotional intelligence:

1. The definition of the concept is constantly changing.
2. Most definitions are so all-inclusive as to make the concept unintelligible.
3. One definition (eg reasoning with emotion) involves a contradiction.
4. There is no such thing as actual emotional intelligence, although intelligence can be applied to emotions as well as to other life domains.

Chapter 6

Models of the medical interview

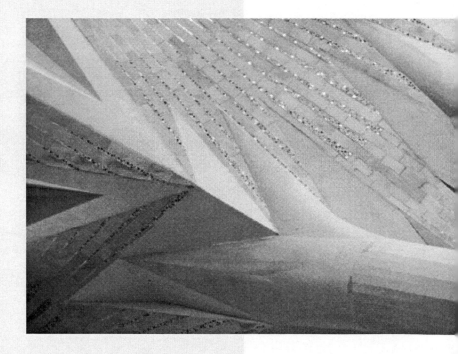

Models of the medical interview

The doctor, the patient and the context

It seems likely that a number of factors influence the choice of career or specialty for doctors, including personality, perceived strengths and weaknesses, and the degree to which a person enjoys communicating and interacting with others. According to Pendleton *et al.* (2003), doctors vary in the amount of emotional involvement they seek or can cope with. MacDonald (2004) explains that 'some of us have an easy open manner and can talk to anyone. Others are more reticent, growing up in families that are more reserved, less extrovert and less expressive. Whatever our background many doctors are reluctant and even fearful to engage with patients.'

Launer (2007) states that: 'of all professions, doctors are invariably the most proficient at not listening. I am struck again and again by how much medical listening – even the kind that sometimes passes for being "patient-centred" – falls desperately short of anything that one might expect from an attentive, untrained friend.'

If this is so, then why are doctors not aware of it? Pendleton *et al.* (2003) suggest that 'the feedback doctors get from their patients is haphazard and unsystematic.' Graugaard & Finset (2000) found that 'even though feedback is not necessarily given to the physician during the consultation, patients will often later express strong emotions about the physician's style of communication.'

There is more happening in the doctor-patient relationship than meets the eye. Both the doctor and the patient are playing or acting out a number of different roles simultaneously. We need to understand these roles in order to become consciously aware of the dynamics of the relationship as they unfold within the consultation. For instance, Roter & Hall (2006) quote research which shows that when doctors liked their patients more, their patients were more satisfied with them (Hall *et al.*, 1993; Hall *et al.*, 2002).

Groopman (2008) writes of Hall's studies of primary care physicians and surgeons:

patients knew remarkably accurately how the doctor actually felt about them. Much of this, of course, comes from nonverbal behaviour: the physician's facial expressions, how he is seated, whether his gestures are warm and welcoming or formal and remote. 'The doctor is supposed to be emotionally neutral and even-handed with everybody,' Hall said, 'and we know that's not true.'

Indeed, 'doctors seem to like their healthier patients more than their less healthy ones' (Hall *et al.*, 1993; Hall *et al.*, 2002 in Roter & Hall, 2006). Roter & Hall (2006) point out that sicker patients behave more negatively (Hall *et al.*, 1996), are likely to be 'grumpy, unresponsive and possibly even unwashed or unkempt and patients whose distress is of an emotional nature may be particularly erratic or unrewarding in interpersonal interaction.'

When patients do not get better, doctors may become frustrated and stop trying (Groopman, 2008); they may feel disappointed, inadequate or angry. Balint said that 'the doctor cannot bear the burden of either not knowing enough or of being unable to help.' Responses to feelings of helplessness and the limitations of medical treatment may include 'rejecting and withdrawing from the patient, blaming the patient for failing to recover, or taking excessive personal responsibility for the patient's failure to recover. Both under- and over-treatment of the patient may ensue' (Turner, 2000).

Salinsky & Sackin (2000) draw attention to the fact that it is important for doctors that 'patients should respond positively to their ministrations.' Groopman (2008) points out the possible consequences if they do not:

Emotion can blur a doctor's ability to listen and think. Physicians who dislike their patients regularly cut them off during the recitation of symptoms and fix on a convenient diagnosis and treatment. The doctor becomes increasingly convinced of the truth of his misjudgement, developing a psychological commitment to it. He becomes wedded to his distorted conclusions. His strong negative feelings about the patient make it harder for him to abandon that conclusion and reframe the clinical picture.

Doctors may have judgmental attitudes about those patients whose lifestyle or behavior has contributed to their disease. Sympathy may be less when harm is perceived to be self-inflicted. Anger and frustration, or an attitude that the patient is therefore less deserving, may be communicated with or without the doctor's conscious awareness.

One man writes:

The most memorable of the consultations with members of the medical profession about my drinking problem.

1. *c. 1971 (21 years old)*

    > Me: *I think I may be drinking too much.*
    > Dr: *Drink less.*

    > *End of conversation.*

2. *c. 1972 (22 years old)*

    > Me: *I'm still drinking too much.*
    > Dr: *Stop drinking.*

    > *End of conversation.*

3. *c. 1983 (33 years old)*

    > Me: *I think I need Antabuse.*
    > Dr: *Fine. (Writes out prescription. End of conversation.)*

4. *c. 1986 (36 years old) (A phone conversation)*

    > Me: *Why have I been refused life insurance?*
    > Dr: *Your medical records show you have a drink problem.*
    > Me: *Do you think it's sensible to penalise drinkers for seeking help?*

    > *(Line goes dead.)*

5.　*c. 1990 (40 years old)*

> Me:　I am obliged to inform you that I'm going into a rehab centre.
>
> Dr:　Would you mind visiting me again when you come out? I've always wanted to know more about those places.

6.　*c. 1995 (45 years old)*

> Me:　I'm an alcoholic. Now in recovery.
>
> Dr:　Why are you telling me that?

Hargie & Dickson (2004), in their skill model of interpersonal communication, described the importance of the person-situation context:

> *What takes place during interaction is partly due to participants and the personal 'baggage' that they bring to the encounter. It includes their knowledge, motives, values, emotions, attitudes, expectations and dispositions… the way in which they have come to regard themselves (self-concept) and the beliefs that they have formed about their abilities to succeed in various types of enterprise (self-efficacy).*

Korsch (1989) writes that 'many authors such as Balint (1964) and Engel (1980) advanced our understanding of the importance of the physicians' personal attitudes about pain, dependence, hostility, noncompliance, poverty, obesity, drugs, homosexuality, and, most of all, about death and dying.' In relation to death, for instance, MacDonald (2004) states that 'a doctor's inability to resolve his own personal experiences of death makes empathy much more difficult and is one of the commonest reasons for doctors to appear cold and unsympathetic.'

It is clear that personal beliefs, attitudes, emotions or experiences in the past or in the present can influence the doctor's emotional response to patients: 'personal experiences in the doctor's life can determine professional actions' (Salinsky & Sackin, 2000). Simply having technical knowledge of diseases does not mean that we have the means of processing the emotions that arise when constantly dealing with people who are sick. Traditionally, doctors have been seen as objective, rational and detached. Yet we know that this is not so. Doctors are human, they are subjective, and they have emotions, which they may express and understand to varying degrees. Salinsky & Sackin (2000) point out that 'we may like to pretend that the "professional self", wearing its physician's white coat, can operate independently of the 'personal self' … the two selves are indivisible, and the defences which spring up to protect our personal feelings will often impair our performance as professionals.'

McWhinney (1989) writes that:

> *All too frequently we do not listen to our patients, perceive their needs, or understand their sufferings. Understanding patients requires in the physician certain personal qualities not usually emphasised in medical education: self-knowledge, moral awareness, a reflective habit of mind, and a capacity for empathy and attentive listening.*

Kurtz *et al.* (2005) quote Epstein (1999) whose view is that 'the block to communication does not lie primarily with poor skills but at a deeper level of attitudes and emotions, of self-awareness and reflection.' Simpson *et al.* (1991) also stress that 'a physician's personal growth and self awareness are essential bases of effective communication.'

Salinsky & Sackin (2000) state that:

> *there are a number of predisposing factors which will make us more likely to avoid subjective encounters with our patients' feelings. These include tiredness, illness, preoccupation with personal problems, anger with colleagues in the practice team and oppression by shortage of time. Perhaps the word 'stress' sums it all up. However, even when not under stress, a consultation can easily suffer from emotional deprivation for other reasons to do with the doctor and/or the patient.*

This chapter looks at some of those other reasons in more depth.

The medical model

In terms of working models, we have already seen that general expectations towards both medicine and doctors are changing. Levenstein *et al.* (1989) emphasise the distinction between 'the disease framework (What is the diagnosis?) and the illness framework (What is the patient's experience of illness: ideas, expectations and feelings?)' The patient-centred or collaborative approach 'involves the patient and the practitioner reaching a mutual understanding of each other's explanatory models of illness and disease' (Griffin *et al.*, 2004). Stewart & Roter (1989) explain that 'physicians bring to medical practice a world view based purely on the biomedical model, which emphasises biochemistry and technology. In contrast, a patient's world comprises a complex web of personality, culture, living situations, and relationships that colour and define the illness experience.'

This description of differing models or world-views has parallels with the concept of schemas. Hargie & Dickson (2004) define the schema as a way of 'explaining how information is organised into a framework representing the world as experienced by the individual and used to interpret current events.' Young *et al.* (2003) explain that 'a schema can be thought of generally as any broad organising principle for making sense of one's life experience.' They describe how 'early maladaptive schemas' arise as a result of childhood experiences, and then maladaptive behaviours develop as responses to these schemas.

For example, if a patient has an inbuilt schema of emotional deprivation, then they will expect that people will not support them or satisfy their needs and that they will let them down. In a medical encounter, then, these feelings may drive behaviour. However the doctor approaches the patient, they are likely to act as if the doctor is not doing enough, that whatever the doctor does is not going to solve the problem, and they might show this through being demanding, unpleasant or hostile. In response to this, the doctor is likely to feel irritated, not particularly sympathetic, and disinclined to do anything more than the bare minimum. If, in addition, the patient's behaviour triggers one of the doctor's own maladaptive schemas, then the doctor may feel inadequate, angry or disproportionately upset, which may lead to showing varying degrees of hostility or disinterest.

In the past, people viewed doctors with awe and respect. More recently, Launer (2007) states that 'fewer and fewer people think that we as doctors can offer them "the truth." Increasingly, they believe that we are offering them one kind of truth among many available... the patients who sit in our waiting rooms are no longer likely to accept that the scientific and medical views of the world trump all others.' Gordon *et al.* (2000) state that the 'illusion of certainty' described by Quill & Suchman (1993) in medicine is now increasingly being replaced – perhaps, as Roter (1989) states, by 'a model of care that values information exchange and shared decision-making over physician certainty and control.'

Maguire (2000) writes that 'patients claim that doctors do not ask them explicitly about their own perceptions of their illness, the prognosis, and related concerns and feelings. Patients also report that doctors do not usually ask them about how they have reacted psychologically to the diagnosis and key treatments, and what the impact has been on their mood, daily lives and personal relationships.' Stewart & Roter (2006) quote a number of studies which confirm this. Their view is that one of the consequences of this 'reluctance to explore how patients perceive their illness and have been affected by it has been that psychiatric morbidity is overlooked in patients (Bridges and Goldberg, 1984; Maguire *et al.*, 1981; Nabarro, 1984; Rosser & Maguire, 1982).'

Maguire (2000) makes the point that:

> *patients who become very distressed and feel that they are struggling to cope with their illness and treatment may be especially loath to admit this to their doctor. They fear that they will be labelled as 'pathetic, inadequate and neurotic.' They also worry that they will be perceived as ungrateful for the care they have been given, and that these judgements will result in their receiving second-class care.*

Turner (2000) quotes several studies which report on the prevalence of affective disorder, which affects 13% of men and 17% of women admitted to general medical wards (Reid *et al.*, 2001); 20–25% of patients with diabetes or rheumatoid arthritis (Fink *et al.*, 1999); and over 30% of acute care admissions and patients with cancer (Hartz *et al.*, 2000). Turner (2000) also points out that 'the families of patients who are chronically ill tend to be more depressed and are more likely to have other psychological symptoms.' Doctors are therefore increasingly called upon to explore emotional and psychological issues with patients although, as Stewart & Roter (2006) point out, 'some doctors are interested only in their patients' physical illnesses and do not want to become embroiled in emotional and social matters.' Patients may also find it very difficult to talk about these issues.

Doctors may expect that patients will tell them 'the whole truth,' or that patients will be able to articulate their problems. In fact, this is often not the case. Hargie & Dickson (2004) state that 'many people have a fear of disclosing too much about their thoughts and feelings, since there is a risk of being rejected, not understood, or subjected to ridicule; causing embarrassment or offence to the listener; or expressing and presenting oneself so badly that a negative image of self is portrayed.'

The biopsychosocial model

George L Engel was dually accredited in medicine and psychiatry, trained in psychoanalysis, and was at the forefront of liaison psychiatry in the 1950s. His paper 'The need for a new medical model: a challenge for biomedicine' was published in 1977, calling for medicine to give 'explicit attention to humanness' (Engel, 1997). When a patient tells their story, they includes thoughts, feelings and associations which allow the doctor to build up a picture of what happened to the patient, and what it meant to them. Engel (2001) points out that this narration of the patient's personal story encourages the development of intimacy within the doctor-patient relationship, and fulfils, for the doctor, the need to know and understand, and, for the patient, the need to feel known and understood, which is a dimension of caring and being cared for.

Engel describes biopsychosocial thinking as providing a conceptual framework for a scientific approach to what patients have to tell us about their illness experiences:

> Feeling 'sick' and 'falling ill' often begin as private experiences not necessarily knowable to anyone else. Hence, the truly scientific

physician not only must access that private world, but also must be reasonably assured that the information (data) accessed can be relied on. Critical is recognition that the patient is both an initiator and a collaborator in the process, not merely an object of study. The physician is a participant observer who, in the process of attending to the patient's reporting of inner-world data, taps into his/her own personal inner viewing system for comparison and clarification. The medium is dialogue, which at various levels includes communing (sharing experiences) as well as communicating (exchanging information). Hence, observation (outer viewing), introspection (inner viewing), and dialogue (interviewing) are the basic methodologic triad for clinical study and for rendering patient data scientific (Engel, 1997).

Smith & Hoppe (1991) explain that:

People are continuously developing a story that portrays what is most important in their lives. The patient's story emerges in a meaningful, integrated, and complete way. The physician's task is to elicit and understand this story, for it provides an introduction to who the person is and why he or she is seeing the physician. The story also provides clues to diagnostic and therapeutic issues relevant to the patient's problem.

The biopsychosocial aspects of the patient-centred method thus include establishing a dialogue, understanding the meaning of the illness for the patient (McWhinney, 1989), and achieving a more humanistic interaction (Smith & Hoppe, 1991). This structure has informed the development of a number of approaches such as the health belief model, motivational interviewing, and techniques for negotiating.

It makes sense that understanding a patient's thoughts and feelings about their illness will inform the doctor of how likely they are to follow advice or a certain treatment plan. Thoughts and perceptions influence actions. For instance, if a patient believes that a particular medication is addictive, then they are not likely to want to take it. It may be that the drug is not addictive, but if the doctor does not elicit this particular belief from the patient, then they will not understand why the drug has not been taken. A patient might believe that a treatment killed their grandmother, and therefore has very negative feelings and associations to that treatment, which need to be understood as only then can they be countered with new information.

Myths and mysteries abound in day to day life. One person said that as a child, one day his grandmother had simply disappeared and no one talked about it. His fantasy was that she had been incarcerated in a mental hospital, but there was also the possibility that she had killed herself. Years later, when he experienced symptoms of anxiety and was referred for a psychiatric assessment, he was terrified that something similar was going to happen to him.

MacDonald (2004) points out that some patients 'may self-diagnose in a way that leads them to have made faulty assumptions. As a result they bring to the consultation a closed mind and the potential for pursuing an entirely faulty approach to their situation.' In other words, a patient's beliefs about their diagnosis and treatment must be assessed, as, without this discussion, the doctor's advice will likely go unheeded.

In terms of influencing or persuading, you have to know what a person believes, and why they believe it, before you can attempt to persuade him to do something else that you think would be better for him. For example, Levinson *et al.* (2001) state that 'one of a physician's most important tasks is to help patients change unhealthy behaviours, such as smoking, hazardous alcohol use, overeating, or physical inactivity. Such lifestyle changes often affect the outcome of care more than any other medical treatments that physicians have to offer.'

The Health Belief Model was first proposed by Rosenstock *et al.* in 1966, and later developed to explain how a patient's beliefs and perceptions affect the likelihood of engaging in treatment, changing lifestyle, or taking preventive measures to protect or improve health.

Ley (1998) explains that the health belief model states that the probability of an individual adopting a health conducive behaviour is affected by that individual's perceptions of:

- Their susceptibility to the illness or danger.
- The severity or seriousness of that illness or danger.
- The effectiveness or benefit of following the recommended course of action.
- The material and psychological costs of, and barriers to, the adoption of the behaviour.

Rollnick *et al.* (2005) state that change is more likely if patients are helped to make decisions for themselves rather than being told what to do:

When practitioners use a directing style, most of the consultation is taken up with informing patients about what the practitioner thinks they should do and why they should do it. When practitioners use a guiding style, they step aside from persuasion and instead encourage patients to explore their motivations and aspirations. The guiding style is more suited to consultations about changing behaviour because it harnesses the internal motivations of the patient. This was the starting point of motivational interviewing.

The concept of motivational interviewing evolved from experience in the treatment of problem drinkers, and was first described by Miller in 1983 and later elaborated by Miller and Rollnick in 1991. According to Rollnick & Miller (1995), it is a directive, client-centred counselling style for eliciting behaviour change by helping clients to explore and resolve ambivalence. It involves:

- Seeking to understand the person's frame of reference, particularly via reflective listening.
- Expressing acceptance and affirmation.
- Eliciting and selectively reinforcing the client's own self motivational statements, expressions of problem recognition, concern, desire and intention to change, and ability to change.
- Monitoring the client's degree of readiness to change, and ensuring that resistance is not generated by jumping ahead of the client.
- Affirming the client's freedom of choice and self-direction.

Levinson *et al.* (2001) outline the stages of change model, which proposes that 'at a specific time, patients are in one of several discrete stages of change:

- Precontemplation;
- Contemplation;
- Determination;
- Action;
- Maintenance; or
- Relapse.

Typically, patients move from one stage to the next as they attempt to change. Relapse into the old unhealthy behavior (for example, smoking) is a common, almost expected, part of the change process.' They explain the different stages for instance in relation to smoking:

> **Precontemplation**: 'I'm not really interested in quitting. It's not a problem.'
>
> Responses: 'I think that the most important thing you can do for your health is to quit smoking.'
>
> 'Could you tell me more about what leads you to feel this way?'
>
> [Build tension between smoking and patient's goals] 'Sounds like you enjoy smoking but also you want good health as you age.'
>
> **Contemplation**: 'I know I should quit, but I really do enjoy smoking. I've got to quit, but with all the stresses in my life right now, I don't know if I can.'
>
> Responses: 'Sounds like you're caught in a bind right now. On one hand, you know that the smoking is bad for your health and you want to quit. On the other hand, you enjoy it because it helps with stress.'
>
> 'Let's look some more at the things you like about smoking and the things you don't like.'
>
> 'I believe you could do this, but I agree that you're not ready to take that step yet.'
>
> **Determination**: 'I have to stop and I'm planning how to do that.'

Responses: 'On a scale of one to ten, how committed are you to quitting?'

'Let's look at the good things that smoking does for you. How will you deal with the absence?'

[Develop an action plan] 'What do you think will work for you? What problems might arise? How will you deal with them?'

Action: 'I'm doing my best. It's tough.'

Responses: 'It's terrific that you want to quit. What's working for you?'

'What problems have you had? How did you solve them?'

'Relapse is common. What will you do should it start to happen?'

Maintenance: 'I've learned a lot through this process.'

Responses: 'What have you learned that helps you continue to avoid cigarettes?'

'Are there situations in which you are tempted to smoke? How do you cope at those times?'

Relapse: 'I blew it.'

Responses: 'I think it's great that you stopped smoking for a period of time.'

'What did you learn that might help you to stop next time?'

'How do you feel about trying again?'

The psychodynamic model

An interesting study was conducted in the U.S. by Melchiode (1979) to determine the role of psychoanalytic concepts in medical education. Questionnaires were sent to directors of medical student education in psychiatry, and it was found that 'practically all of the sixty-six respondents indicated that psychodynamic theory had been incorporated into major required courses. More than half considered the concepts of defence mechanism, countertransference, transference, and dynamic unconscious necessary to general education.'

So what can we learn from a psychoanalytical approach?

In psychoanalysis, consideration of transference and countertransference is central to the analysis. Within the relationship between therapist and client, feelings arise toward each other that derive from past relationships. These feelings are projected onto the other person as though that person has 'caused' them, whereas in fact the person has simply triggered feelings from another time and place that were already there. This means that the examination of the feelings that the patient feels towards the therapist are vital in understanding what his past relationships have been like. For instance, a patient may have suffered harsh and critical treatment by a parent, and if the therapist says something that the patient interprets as being in any way critical, the therapist has become the critical parent in the patient's eyes, and they react to the therapist with whatever feelings were aroused in that relationship. These feelings might be of rage or hopelessness or depression. Whatever feelings are aroused in the patient, they may have a force and vehemence which can be surprising to the patient. The therapist reflects with him or her on the meaning of their feelings, and memories often arise of occasions on which the patient experienced similar emotions at other times their. The therapist makes the link between the past emotional events and the present day feelings. This process of experiencing, reflecting, and gaining insight continues throughout the therapy. It means that powerful emotions can be examined to shed light on the patient's early relationships and experiences.

It is interesting that various pointers to a person's past traumatic emotions have arisen in the therapy not through talking but through experiencing and analysing the transference. Freud, the founder of psychoanalysis, writes that the patient 'is repeating before our eyes his old defensive actions; he would like best to repeat in his relation to the analyst all the history of that forgotten period of his life. So what he is showing us is the kernel of his intimate life history: he is reproducing it tangibly, as though it were actually happening, instead of remembering it.' As Sloane (1993) writes, transference is 'the repetition and reworking in the present of painful patterns of experience that had their origins in past relationships.' For Corradi (2006), it is 'the tendency to repeat formative human relationships in later life, and is a universal developmental characteristic.'

The psychoanalytic or psychotherapeutic situation is different to most other therapeutic relationships in that the therapist or analyst has undergone their own analysis. This means that they have become aware of the origins of their strong emotional reactions to situations and have acknowledged and made sense of their own early experiences. Thus when the patient starts to project feelings onto them, they do not respond automatically with feelings such as anger, defensiveness or hostility. Sometimes the patient's behaviour does provoke these responses from people in their life, with whom they have relationships, as they are not aware of this mechanism of projection. But the behaviours and feelings that the patient exhibits in therapy sessions are not judged or responded to emotionally by the therapist. This is one of the most vitally important functions of the relationship – for new learning to occur through relationship. The patient learns that the therapist treats them with kindness, compassion and understanding, and will work with them to understand and resolve their inner conflicts and problems. In this way, the wounds of the past can be examined and made sense of within the safe and nurturing environment of the relationship.

The importance of the relationship cannot be overemphasised. Indeed, Carotenuto & Tambureno (1991) state that 'movement toward healing is not possible without the medium of relationship, created by the interacting personalities of analyst and analysand.' Corradi (2006) states that 'when patients experience a relationship in which a mature, caring person with no personal axe to grind listens to them and takes them seriously, tacitly gives them permission to be autonomous and pursue self-fulfilling goals, or serves as an exemplary role model eliciting identification, these corrective emotional experiences can change peoples' lives.'

Interestingly, there are many parallels with the relationship between patient and doctor. Sloane (1993) states that 'all patients, whether in psychotherapy or in surgery, project onto the person of the doctor their deepest hopes and darkest fears.' Blum (1985) writes that 'in the relationship between physician and patient certain phenomena occur that are comparable to responses in the relationship between the psychoanalyst and analysand, such as transference and countertransference. This indicates that the physician in physical health care in effect is involved in some kind of psychotherapy.' This means that we can use our emotional responses to other people, whether patients or otherwise, as a means of understanding more about ourselves and about them.

According to Freud (1997: 1910), 'transference arises spontaneously in all human relationships.' The importance of early childhood experiences is emphasised as this is the place where emotional responses first occurred and patterns were started which continue into adulthood. All of us learned the world from our parents or first caregivers. We copied their ways of dealing with their emotions because we were unaware of any alternatives, and we learned from how they acted, not from any stated guidance – so we might have learned to withdraw and sulk when angry, or to shout and become aggressive when upset, or to react to disappointment by becoming depressed.

For example:

> When I was about six years old, my mother used to bang the cutlery into the drawer when she was angry, and if asked what the matter was, would dissolve into tears and be completely unable to articulate what she was feeling. It would therefore come as no surprise that as a young adult, I would allow anger to build and build, then finally it would explode and I would feel so overwhelmed by emotion that I would not be able to say rationally what was upsetting me, but would start to cry. To be aware of those patterns is not a question of disloyalty to parents, or apportioning blame, or judging them or me, it is rather a means of working out what emotional blueprints I did learn, and whether they now serve me.

Freud wrote: 'it is only experiences in childhood that explain susceptibility to later traumas and it is only by uncovering these almost invariably forgotten memory-traces and by making them conscious that we acquire the power to get rid of the symptoms.' The symptoms might be lack of assertiveness, avoidance of conflict, difficulty expressing feelings, problems with intimacy or trust, low self-esteem, problems with temper ... the list goes on. Almost everyone displays these at one time or another. If many problems coexist, constellations of symptoms may produce physical or psychological symptoms which then come to be regarded as an illness.

Freud found that unpleasant or traumatic emotions in childhood come to be repressed, that is, pushed out of the conscious mind, because they are difficult to bear. They are stored as memories, images, emotions in the unconscious mind, and the stronger the repression, the less likely that the person can bring them voluntarily to conscious awareness. They are, in effect, buried but not dead. To the small child, the world is big, emotions threaten to overwhelm, and resources to cope with them are few. Therefore all sorts of experiences may have provoked fear, anxiety, sadness, anger, which to the child seemed unbearably intense and which therefore threatened his or her sense of security and self. Because they are unpleasant, the person does not want to remember these memories. When they are remembered, the emotion is the big emotion of the small child, and therefore seems not only intensely powerful but also irrational to the adult who is experiencing them. For this reason, we resist consciously bringing such material to mind.

Freud writes: 'Resistance finds it easy to disguise itself as an intellectual rejection... The arrogance of consciousness (in rejecting dreams with such contempt, for instance) is one of the most powerful of the devices with which we are provided as a universal protection against the incursion of unconscious complexes.'

Delaney (2007) writes:

> *Repressed experiences are stronger than reason or argument or cognitive therapy; willy-nilly they are enacted again and again in many different ways and in many different settings throughout the patient's life, unless and until the intolerable repressed feelings and their triggering events have been identified, consciously experienced, and reacted to (with sadness, anger or indignation) by the sufferer. The only way this can be done is for the patient to revisit them: if all else fails, alone; but let's hope she can do so in the company of someone willing to listen, during some form of 'talking' therapy.*

The psychodynamics of the doctor-patient relationship

Corradi (2006) explains that:

> *through transference, patients bring to the physician feelings, attitudes, and behaviours that belonged to childhood parental figures. This is a process facilitated by the physician's authority and by regressive feelings of dependency often associated with being ill. Transference attitudes may quickly show themselves, often through exaggerated behaviours, for example, diffidence, over-familiar or ingratiating attitudes, defensive or hostile withholding, and attempts to control the interview.*

For example, if the patient enters the encounter with feelings of aggression and hostility towards the doctor as a transference of the feelings of aggression and hostility that they felt towards their parents in childhood, then if the doctor understands the origin of those feelings, they do not have to respond automatically. The doctor can then observe what is happening without their own emotional response getting in the way. If the doctor is not aware of the transference, then they will automatically react with their own countertransference.

Countertransference is the doctor's emotional response to the patient. The patient may behave in such as way as to induce in the doctor those very feelings they are experiencing, such as anxiety, irritation, anger, hopelessness, helplessness, or desperation. If the doctor is aware of these feelings as they arise, they can give valuable information about the patient's mental state. They are in effect feeling the emotion that the patient cannot articulate. If the doctor is not aware of the true origin of these feelings, then they simply react automatically to them.

Klyman *et al.* (2008) state that the relevance of understanding transference is to help the doctor to 'understand the common dynamics of the doctor-patient relationship; to understand the psychological aspects of various physical symptoms; and manage challenging patients to optimize their quality of life, cost-effectiveness of treatment and minimize physician burnout.' They point out that:

some patients are unable to participate in a good, mutually cooperative relationship with their primary care doctors. They may have long-standing psychosocial difficulties exacerbated by chronic, painful, or life-threatening illnesses. Some may have somatic symptoms that they define as evidence only of an identified illness but which are reflections of psychic misery with roots in their thoughts, feelings, and relationships.

Mollon (2001) points out that at least one third of consultations in primary care involve psychological problems:

The GP's work is pervaded by psychological dimensions and emotional pain, even when the presenting problem is not overtly a mental disorder ... Illness evokes anxieties and confusions that are both infantile and unconscious. The patient's emotional relationship with their GP is infiltrated by transference based on their infantile relationship with parents. The GP must be open to the communication of emotional pain, modelled on the child's plea seeking of reassurance from a parent, whilst also able to withstand the danger of being affectively overwhelmed.

Strous *et al.* (2006) report that 'physicians may encounter a subset of patients who engender strong negative feelings, despair and even downright malice.' These patients have been called 'heart-sink' or 'hateful' patients. Delaney (2007) suggests that:

we could see the 'heart-sink' patient as someone for whom things went seriously wrong early on in life: in a relationship of trust, at a vulnerable stage in development. Our difficulty in 'getting the picture' may indicate we are dealing with a patient's repressed experience, re-enacted in exact but obscure ways, using the listener/ doctor as a ready-to-hand and convenient figure of transference.

Sloane (1993) states that these enactments 'may result in the therapist feeling injured or unfairly blamed, sexually or aggressively aroused, anxious, ashamed or guilty.' Delaney (2007) explains that in any given consultation, the patient:

may allocate the role of the child to himself, casting the listener as the unsatisfactory adult. Or the patient may keep the role of the all-powerful adult for himself and relieve his old feelings of pain, humiliation and incomprehension by attempting to inflict them

on the listener, so that the doctor is cast as the former child. The listener's feelings, of anger and irritation, elicited in response to such a consultation, are the feelings the patient may have experienced in a long-past but crucial relationship or situation.

It can be very difficult for the doctor to deal with this, especially if they doe not understand the reasons for it happening. Sloane (1993) points out that some patients 'need to make their doctor suffer and even drive him or her "crazy"' – in effect so that the doctor knows firsthand how the patient has suffered in the past in their early relationships.'

Balint (1957) points out that 'if the doctor understands the pattern and can demonstrate it convincingly to his patient, the rigidity of the repetition loosens up and something else may happen.' Matthews *et al.* (1993) quote Hiatt (1986), who states that 'the patient's unconscious process is our most important resource, provided we are alert to its methods of expression. Unconscious process will persistently urge the patient toward healing and growth and attempt to bring underlying problems to light, within the bounds of what the patient can accept consciously.'

By not simply reacting to the patient's projections, but by listening and providing a supportive relationship, the doctor gives the patient an opportunity to move on from those old patterns. Launer (2007) states that:

> *whether this relationship lasts for a single medical consultation, or a long course of therapy, it may help to correct some of the hurt done by less well-attuned relationships, or by significant losses and setbacks, and to make sense of them. What is particularly interesting is that a growing amount of collaborative research, done by neuroscientists and psychiatrists working together, suggests that such processes may bring about demonstrable changes at a neurological level (Kaplan-Solms & Solms, 2000).*

The holistic model

The Royal College of Physicians (2005) state that 'well-being indicates the holistic notion of achieving a state of health, comfort and happiness. It encompasses the physical, mental, and social aspects of a patient's life, aspects that the doctor seeks to heal or repair.' Dixon *et al.* (1999) write that 'it is clear that the art of healing and the strength of the doctor-patient relationship play a vital role in improving the well-being of patients.'

Stewart (2005) suggests that doctors need 'an awareness of the whole person in context, that is an awareness of the multiple aspects of the patient's life.' Her view is that 'current societal values do not, on the whole, support or nurture relationship.'

Reynolds & Scott (2000) observe that:

> *the low level of empathy observed in psychologists, nurses, occupational therapists and doctors should be a serious concern to those professional groups and to educators. As research shows a positive relationship between professional empathy and outcome, the low level of empathy reported across all professions indicates that many professional helpers are simply not as helpful as they ought to be.*

Indeed, DiMatteo & Taranta (1979) quote Cobb who found as far back as 1954 that 'lack of physician-patient rapport often forces chronically and terminally ill patients to seek help and understanding from nonmedical healers.'

Mercer *et al.* (2001) state that 'the call to integrate complementary treatments into the NHS is one issue, but the organisational, structural, and personal limitations that general practitioners and hospital specialists in conventional medicine face in trying to provide holistic care is a wider one. Needing to prove that compassion is not a luxury but a fundamental requirement of a healthcare system is a damning indictment of our current ways of thinking.' Abramovitch & Schwartz (1996) state that 'the negative consequences of physicians' failure to establish and maintain personal relationships with patients are at the heart of the "humanistic crisis" in medicine.'

DiMatteo & Taranta (1979) found in the 'medical, public health, and social-psychological literature strong indications of the critical importance of supplementing the technical knowledge and expertise of physicians with effective interpersonal treatment. The literature was replete with evidence that the process by which healing takes place is, in part, an interpersonal one.' And yet, as Weston & Lipkin (1989) comment:

> *young physicians may have a staggering knowledge of disease but be naïve about human suffering; they may know precise drug treatment but stand empty-handed and mute before the patient who desperately needs counsel and support to cope with a terminal illness; they may be masters of medicine's remarkable biotechnical resources but lack power to heal the human spirit.*

So what is healing? The words health, healing and holistic all come from the same Germanic root, whole. As Dosanjh *et al.* (2001) point out, 'intuitively people know that health has to do with wholeness.' McWhinney (1989) states that 'healing is not the same as treating or curing.' Matthews *et al.* (1993) write that 'healers must try to understand what the illness means to the patient and create a therapeutic sense of connection in the patient-clinician relationship.' They describe 'connexional moments' in which doctor and patient share understanding and experience a transpersonal or spiritual dimension. 'These moments are often marked by a physiologic reaction, such as gooseflesh or a chill; by an immediacy of awareness of the patient's situation (as if experiencing it from inside the patient's world); by a sense of being part of a larger whole; and by a lingering feeling of joy, peacefulness, or awe.' They quote a number of studies which report that 'such moments seem to be therapeutic for the patient and the clinician alike (Suchman & Matthews, 1988; Branch & Suchman, 1990; Suchman *et al.*, 1993).'

Travaline *et al.* (2005) believe that medical encounters involve:

> *the patient's search for a psychosocial healing 'connexion,' or therapeutic relationship. For example, a patient with broken relationships with family, friends, co-workers, or the community in general, will often struggle when describing his illness and symptoms for the first time. That patient's contact with his physician is often a first step toward reconnection. Therefore, it is essential for the physician to listen to patient concerns, provide comfort and healing, and foster the relationship in general.*

Egnew's view (2009) is that 'physician-healers use the power of the doctor-patient relationship to help patients discover or create new illness narratives with fresh meanings that reconnect them to the world and to others and thereby transcend suffering and experience healing.'

Longhurst (1989) states that:

> *Traditionally, the power of the healer was the catalyst in the therapeutic relationship. The healing effect of that power came from a conscious (or unconscious) willingness of a patient to believe that the healer, through science, intent, energy and creativity would bring a reintegration of the troubled person. The most powerful healers had special qualities: an enhanced ability to induce an altered state of consciousness and an adeptness at controlling the expression of 'healing energy.'*

Longhurst (1989) quotes Howard Stein (1985) who said of the physician self, 'one can truly recognise a patient only if one is willing to recognise oneself in the patient.' Longhurst goes on to consider the question of whether one needs to be a 'wounded healer' to be a true physician:

> *Many people believe so: 'he cannot heal until he has healed himself' (Pellegrino, 1983); 'learn that for a physician, healing of yourself takes place through the healing of others' (Tumulty, 1978); 'the healer undertakes to heal himself, to become a whole person … as a first step he accepts and "owns" his powers and potentials and, specifically, his own limitations' (De Vries, 1985).*

Perez (2004) notes that 'research articles and writings have appeared addressing the spiritual dimension of healing (the art of medicine), which often ignored creates a gap in the medical care of the patient. The spiritual aspects of medical care include: communication (listening, speaking), connection (space, safety, and sacredness), and communion through which healing can occur.'

Chapter 7

Barriers to communication

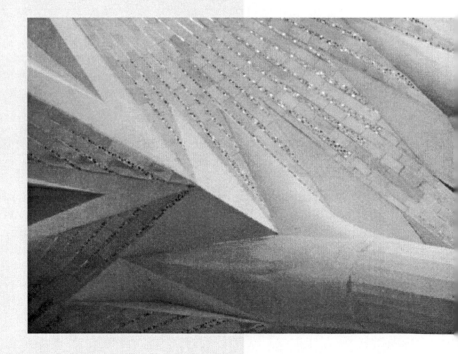

Barriers to communication

Racial and cultural differences

Tomorrow's Doctors (GMC, 2003) states that graduates must be able to do the following:

- Communicate effectively with individuals regardless of their social, cultural or ethnic backgrounds, or their disabilities.
- Communicate with individuals who cannot speak English, including working with interpreters.

Pena Dolhun *et al.* (2003) explain that medical education is responding to an increasingly diverse population by developing cross-cultural curricula:

> *This undertaking has proved problematic because there is no consensus on what elements of cross-cultural medicine should be taught. Further, less is known about what is being taught. A total of 19 medical schools supplied their curricular materials. There was considerable variation in approaches to teaching and in the content of cross cultural education across the schools. Most emphasized teaching general themes, such as the doctor-patient relationship, socioeconomic status, and racism. Most also focused on specific cultural information about the ethnic communities they served. Few schools extensively addressed health care access and language issues.*

Good communication depends upon the ability to understand and be understood. If a patient has poor English language skills, many misunderstandings may arise. These may be avoided by the patient being accompanied by a relative or friend who is able to speak English, but this may present problems in terms of how much sensitive information the patient is likely to divulge in such a situation. Professional interpreters are available and can be arranged to attend at the medical interview. Most are excellent and helpful. However, in a small minority community, it may be that the interpreter already knows the patient socially, and this may lead to a patient being reluctant to give intimate personal details. Or, as Launer (2007) states: 'I found all sorts of deviances between the patients' utterances and what the interpreters conveyed. The interpreters were pretty selective in what they wanted the doctor to know, and occasionally even berated patients for apparent inconsistencies.'

Ferguson & Candib (2002) report research which shows that professional interpreters do help non-English speaking patients to access health services, although they point out that 'at least one study demonstrated persistently poor communication skills on the part of the physicians using such interpreters.' Lack of time can be an issue which leads to physician frustration or empathy failure, as it usually takes about twice as long to interview a patient using an interpreter.

A further issue is that not all doctors are fully proficient in English. As pointed out by the BMA (2004), 'doctors who qualify within the European Economic Area (EAA) do not need to take a language test' GMC (2002). They are therefore able to practise in the UK when their language skills may in fact be problematic.

But language is only one of the barriers which emerge in cross-cultural medical communication studies. Karel (2007) points out that:

> *cultural attitudes, beliefs, and practices − related to racial, ethnic, religious, regional, and other influences − inform all aspects of medical decision making. Culture informs beliefs about the meanings, causes, and cures of illness; what or who can help when illness strikes; as well as who should be involved in making decisions about medical care (eg the patient, family, community, doctor, and/or other healers).*

Schouten & Meeuwesen (2006) outlined five key predictors of culture-related communication problems which had been identified in the literature:

1. Cultural differences in explanatory models of health and illness;
2. Differences in cultural values;
3. Cultural differences in patients' preferences for doctor-patient relationships;
4. Racism/perceptual biases;
5. Linguistic barriers.

Ferguson & Candib (2002) conducted a literature review which found consistent evidence that:

> *race, ethnicity, and language have substantial influence on the quality of the doctor patient relationship. Minority patients, especially those not proficient in English, are less likely to engender empathic response from physicians, establish rapport with physicians, receive sufficient information, and be encouraged to participate in medical decision making.*

Bruijnzeels & Visser (2005) state that 'many researchers argue that ethnic differences between both parties are a potential cause for misunderstanding and lead to a loss of quality of care.' They reason that problems arise as a result of the 'differences in a whole set of values, norms, attitudes and expectations of the patient and the doctor before they meet each other.' Schouten & Meeuwesen (2007) also report that 'consultations of ethnic-minority patients tend to result in poor mutual understanding between doctor and patient, which may have serious consequences for health care.'

Schouten & Meeuwesen (2006) state that culture and ethnicity have often been cited as barriers in establishing an effective and satisfying doctor-patient relationship. They conducted a literature review which revealed:

> *major differences in doctor-patient communication as a consequence of patients' ethnic backgrounds. Doctors behave less affectively when interacting with ethnic minority patients compared to White patients. Ethnic minority patients themselves are also less verbally expressive; they seem to be less assertive and affective during the medical encounter than White patients.*

It is therefore not surprising to find that many ethnic minority patients prefer to see a doctor of the same ethnic origin. In the United States, Gray & Stoddard (1997) found that 'minority patients are significantly more likely to report having a minority physician as their regular doctor. We estimate that minority patients are five times as likely as non-minorities to report that their regular physician is a member of a racial/ethnic minority. This effect is especially pronounced among Hispanics.' Ferguson & Candib (2002) state that 'some of the literature also validates calls for a more diverse physician workforce, since minority patients are more likely to choose minority physicians, be more satisfied by language-concordant relationships, and feel more connected and involved in decision making with racially concordant physicians.' However, not all studies support these findings. Shah & Ogden (2006) report that 'a doctor's age and gender have a stronger impact on a patient's judgements than their ethnicity.'

The important point is that every patient is an individual and even though they may belong to a particular racial or ethnic group, you cannot make assumptions about what that means to that individual.

Coulehan *et al.* (2001) suggest guidelines for clinical empathy in the cross-cultural setting:

- Understand your own cultural values and biases.
- Develop a familiarity with the cultural values, health beliefs, and illness behaviours of ethnic, cultural, and religious groups served in your practice.
- Ask how the patient prefers to be addressed.
- Determine the patient's level of fluency in English and arrange for a translator, if needed.
- Assure the patient of confidentiality; rumours, jealousy, privacy, and reputation are crucial issues in close-knit traditional communities.
- Use a speech rate, tone, and style that promote understanding and show respect for the patient.
- Check back frequently to determine patient understanding and acceptance.

The balance of power

Goodyear-Smith & Buetow (2001) state that:

> *power is an inescapable aspect of all social relationships, and inherently is neither good nor evil. Doctors need power to fulfil their professional obligations to multiple constituencies including patients, the community and themselves. Patients need power to formulate their values, articulate and achieve health needs, and fulfil their responsibilities. However, both parties can use or misuse power.*

Extensive empirical data and theory describe the inequality of power in relations between doctors and their patients (Salmon & May, 1995). Charles *et al.* (2000) point out that 'typically, doctors have more power than patients to structure the nature of the interaction between them. As a consequence, patients may feel that their voice is overridden, silenced, or stripped of personal meaning and social context.'

Being ill can be painful, unpleasant and anxiety-provoking. It generally means that patients are less able than usual to concentrate and take in information. They may be confused by the complexity, terminology, and technology of medicine. Patients may feel as if they are being treated like children, and they often regress to a lower level of functioning than usual. Bub (2006) states that 'illness and engagement with the healthcare system strip power away from the typical patient. The entire environment is unfamiliar, intimidating, and frightening, especially as patients are dependent on others for guidance and help.'

If, in addition to this, doctors make decisions about treatment and management without negotiating with the patient and arriving at an agreement, then misunderstandings arise (Britten *et al.*, 2000); patients are less compliant with medicines (Charles *et al.*, 2000); and patients are less satisfied if doctors are more dominant (Roter & Hall, 2006).

Various approaches to decision-making in medicine have been described, including the paternalistic, the shared and the informed approach. The paternalistic approach involves eliciting physical symptoms and then the doctor making a diagnosis. 'In the "pure type" of this approach doctors can then make a treatment decision that they think is in their patients' best interest without having to explore each patient's values and concerns' (Charles *et al.*, 2000). Kaplan *et al.* (1989) suggest that 'it is possible that doctors are more controlling with (ie ask more questions of, interrupt more often, are more directive with), and therefore less prone to provide information to, sicker patients.' While in certain circumstances this may be understandable in that the acutely sick patient may be less able or unable to take part in the decision-making process, it is also possible that doctors tend to favour a particular approach across a variety of situations rather than adapt themselves to each individual circumstance.

Charles *et al.* (2000) state that:

> *in the informed approach patients are accorded a more active role in both defining the problem for which they want help and in determining appropriate treatment. In the pure type of this approach the doctor's role is limited to providing relevant research information about treatment options and their benefits and risks so that the patient can make an informed decision.*

However, MacDonald (2004) makes the point that 'citing research work and statistics can be extremely intimidating for the patient and create the impression for some patients that the doctor is "coercing" the patient into receiving the whole series of treatments.' It can be very difficult for patients to understand the concepts of relative risk and to see their own individual situation in the context of statistics and probabilities, especially when they are feeling anxious.

In the shared approach, 'doctors commit themselves to an interactive relationship with patients in developing a treatment recommendation that is consistent with patient values and preferences' (Charles *et al.*, 2000).

'If the diagnosis and treatment are seen as the doctor's alone, then adherence is likely to be poor' (Pendleton *et al.*, 2003). Involving patients in the decision in the consultation leads to increased adherence afterwards (Brody *et al.*, 1989).

Pendleton *et al.* (2003) take the view that authoritarian consulting styles tend not to work:

> *The style of consulting that works most effectively is one in which patients are fully involved in all aspects – including diagnosis and decisions about the management of the problem. Patients tend to disregard or minimise the significance of general explanations and advice. They pay more attention to, and follow through with, advice that is believed to be for them personally.*

Pendleton *et al.* (2003) quote Smith *et al.* (1994) who suggest that the patient wants to 'feel that the doctor knows him as a person, and explains the treatment decisions with this personal knowledge in mind.'

Goodyear-Smith & Buetow (2001) state that:

> *the ethical effectiveness of a health system is maximised by empowering doctors and patients to develop 'adult-adult' rather than 'adult-child' relationships that respect and enable autonomy, accountability, fidelity and humanity. Even in adult-adult relationships, conflicts and complexities arise. Lack of concordance between doctors and patients can encourage paternalism but may be best resolved through negotiated care.*

The doctor-patient relationship is central to medical practice, but it constitutes only one part of the system that supports and defines it. In reality, the balance of power is presently changing. Edwards *et al.* (2002) write of 'the growing use of guidelines, protocols, audit, regulation and inspection that many doctors perceive as eroding their control over their professional lives.' Transparency and accountability feature much more prominently than in past times. Furthermore, 'the easy availability of health information coupled with a sense of entitlement is shifting the power in the doctor-patient relationship and causing unease. The job is difficult and emotionally demanding and doctors are more likely to be self critical and have other personality traits associated with work related stress' (Edwards *et al.*, 2002).

Attitudes

It has been noted that some doctors show 'a lack of inclination to communicate with patients' (BMA, 2004).

Roter & Hall (2006) report a study by Kramer *et al.* (1997) who found that skills training to increase self awareness and sensitivity to patients substantially reduced the levels of negativity shown by both medical students and doctors up to a year afterwards, whereas the control group actually increased their use of rejecting behaviours over time. 'Rejecting behaviour included sarcasm, contempt, verbal rejection, non-responsiveness to the patient's statement and evading eye contact.' Weston & Lipkin (1989) quote a memorable example: 'In would sweep twelve coats, never introduce themselves, discourse loudly over the bed in technical jargon, then sweep out without a word.'

MacDonald (2004) makes the point that 'some doctors just don't think that what patients have to say is of much interest. Herein lies the first step on a perilous path to arrogance and a catalogue of complications.' Zoppi & Epstein (2002) state that 'fatigue, dogmatism, unexamined negative emotions, and an overemphasis on behaviour (rather than on self-awareness) may close the mind to ideas and feelings and diminish the possibility of forming a relationship (Epstein, 1999).'

For example, Wileman *et al.* (2002) state that:

> *GPs often call into question the legitimacy of patients presenting with physical symptoms unrelated to organic pathology. Such consultations were frustrating for the GP and potentially harmful to the patient. Patients with medically unexplained symptoms were seen to be presenting with inappropriate symptoms that were a manifestation of emotional or social distress. GPs felt ill-equipped to deal with the presentations and the frustrations they felt.*

Kurtz *et al.* (2005) argue that 'the acquisition of skills can open the path to changes in attitude.' However, Salinsky & Sackin (2000) take the view that it may be necessary for doctors in training 'to be helped to acquire greater self-awareness. Our impression is that with current methods not enough attention is paid to the doctor's own feelings.' As Bub (2006) states, 'emotional health is greatest when knowledge (intellect) and feeling (emotion) are cultivated and integrated rather than separated. Many people spend years in psychotherapy trying to accomplish this. The culture of medicine encourages the opposite.'

Chochinov (2007) emphasises the need for healthcare providers:

> *to examine their attitudes and assumptions towards patients. Attitude can be defined as an enduring, learnt predisposition to behave in a consistent way towards a given class of objects (or people) ... not as they are but as they are conceived to be.*

Chochinov (2007) suggests a list of questions for doctors to ask themselves:

- How would I be feeling in this patient's situation?
- What is leading me to draw those conclusions?

- Have I checked whether my assumptions are accurate?
- Am I aware how my attitude towards the patient may be affecting him or her?
- Could my attitude towards the patient be based on something to do with my own experiences, anxieties, or fears?
- Does my attitude towards being a healthcare provider enable or disenable me to establish open and empathic professional relationships with my patients?

Time constraints

The BMA (2004) describes various organisational barriers to effective communication: 'work constraints include lack of time, pressure of work, and interruptions. These are often symptoms of wider organisational problems that are beyond the doctor's direct control. For example, when an emphasis is placed on "patient throughput," time given to communicating with patients may not be given a high priority.'

Shortage of time can put the doctor under pressure. Salinsky & Sackin (2000) state that this can prevent a doctor from feeling available to share and experience the patient's feelings: 'if a consultation goes on too long, he begins to feel symptoms of panic. His defences click into place and he becomes impervious to the effects of the patient's emotions.'

Sometimes a patient will say something important or start to get upset right at the end of a consultation. The doctor has the choice whether to ask the patient to book another appointment and talk about it then, or to give the patient extra time which means that they run over time throughout his clinic or surgery. Salinsky & Sackin (2000) take the view that it is best not to put the patient off till another time as:

> he may be just at the point where his need to be heard has become critical. He may have been trying to get up courage for some time, he may have been waiting several days already for an appointment with the doctor he knows and trusts. Something already said in the consultation may have released some deep feelings and made the tears start to flow. So it is better to sit back and give the patient at least another ten minutes.

It is important to give the patient the sense that although they have been upset, and some difficult emotions have been released, there will be time to speak again. You might want to say something like: 'I know that this has been hard today, but it's good that you have been able to tell me what you've been feeling. Generally feelings only come to mind when we are able to deal with them. I guess you've been thinking about saying something for some time.' The patient will then see that you do recognise that they have been struggling with some difficult issues, and they may feel a sense of relief that these have finally been articulated.

After patients have become upset, it is helpful to tell them that they are likely to feel drained or fragile for some hours. Emotion is hard work, so it is sensible for them to be gentle with themselves and to give themselves time to get back into balance. Closing the session in this way reassures the patient that it is ok to have felt how they did, and also shows that you are looking after them and helping them to contain their emotions until the next time.

Chapter 8

Healing through relationship

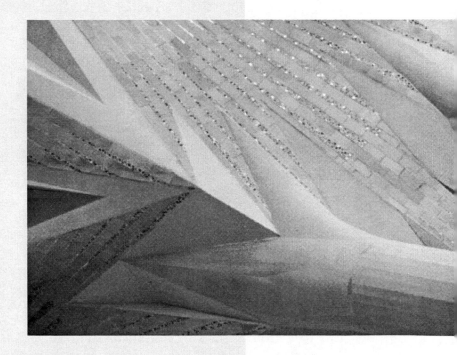

Healing through relationship

The value of the holistic approach

One woman writes:

> At seventeen years old, I developed a painful lump in my breast.
> I saw a young female doctor at my local surgery who told me to
> come back in a week if it was no better. She gave me no indication
> as to what it might be, or how it might develop. Being only
> seventeen, I did as I was told and asked no questions. In exactly
> one week I returned. The 'lump' was now rock hard, very angry
> and extremely painful. I saw an older doctor; a man known for his
> brusque manner. He terrified me. He told me to undress in a side
> room, took a brief look at me, grunted and walked out. I sat on the
> bed, scared to move. I heard him pick up the phone and say: 'Get
> me the hospital.' I waited, shivering. A few minutes later he came
> back in, looked me up and down and said: 'Get dressed.'

> By the time I went through to his room, he was on the phone
> again. He was saying: 'I don't want an appointment next week, I
> need it now.' His urgency frightened me. The phone call finished,
> he made a few notes, and said 'You'll need to go to Outpatients at
> the Royal Infirmary on Friday, reception will give you the details.'
> I left, confused and upset. He had not made eye contact with me
> once. I phoned the surgery the next day in tears. I had no idea
> where the Infirmary was, let alone how to get there. All attempts
> I had made to find someone to take me had failed. An ambulance
> was organised.

> On the Friday, I saw a young Asian doctor. He didn't tell me his
> name. A nurse was with me. He looked at my breast and said: 'Have
> you done anything that might have caused this?' I was stunned,
> I had no idea what might have caused it. He didn't wait for an
> answer. He said to the nurse: 'Get me an anaesthetist,' turned
> on his heel, and, as he was leaving the room, added, 'And make
> it snappy, I'm off at four.' I was left feeling that I had obviously
> created this myself and was a nuisance to everyone. I was put into
> a curtained off area of a room with just a single metal chair. In the
> next curtained off area were two middle-aged women discussing
> their previous operations. One part of their conversation has

stayed in my memory for thirty-three years: 'The worst one I ever had was the one on my breast. That was terrible.' I was shaking so much the chair was rattling. When I was finally called, a big, black woman, presumably the anaesthetist, helped me to climb on to the bed. I was too frightened to cry. She said incredulously to the doctor: 'This child is terrified, she's shaking like a leaf.' She was kind. The doctor looked but said nothing.

I awoke on a bed in a corridor. People were passing by as I tried to make sense of what was happening. Eventually I asked a young nurse what I should do. She said she didn't know and maybe I should ask at reception. Groggy from the general anaesthetic, and still wearing only a theatre gown, I walked out into A&E reception and asked if I could leave. The answer was: 'Who are you?' On making some enquiries, the receptionist then informed me that as far as the hospital was concerned, I had been discharged hours ago. I spent another half an hour wandering around asking people if they knew where my clothes were. Nobody told me what had been done to me and when I asked subsequently, I was told my notes had been lost.

Seventeen years later, I was having another breast 'lump' investigated. Older, wiser and a lot more assertive, I refused to accept everything unquestioningly, and was labelled 'difficult.' A thinly veiled threat was made to withdraw access to treatment unless I just did as I was told! When I pointed this out, I was passed on to a young registrar. He addressed me by my name, listened attentively while I told him my history, and kept eye contact with me whilst he said how sorry he was for the experience I'd had. He then explained to me the procedure that I'd had seventeen years previously. It's difficult to understand how it took me so long to find a doctor worthy of the title.

In this instance, the pain of the past was eased by concern and understanding in the present. The doctor took her seriously, explained things clearly, and expressed regret for the unpleasantness of her previous experiences.

Sometimes doctors seem to forget how frightening not only illness but treatment and the whole hospital experience can be. Richards (1990) makes the point that 'even the briefest spell on the other side of the desk or in a hospital bed gives blinding insight into patients' vulnerability and of their need to be listened to, treated with respect, and given full, unhurried, jargon free explanations. Simple gestures of kindness and encouragement go a long way – as does the occasional admission of fallibility.'

A variety of authors have described aspects of the therapeutic relationship including: listening to patient concerns; providing comfort and healing (Matthews *et al.*, 1993; Suchman & Matthews 1988 in Travaline *et al.*, 2005); sharing experiences ('been through a lot together') (Mainous *et al.*, 2004 in Stewart, 2004); upholding patients' sense of dignity and affirming their value: 'seeing the person they are or were, rather than just the illness they have' (Chochinov, 2007).

Sometimes, however, there simply is no relationship. One woman writes: 'I am having a hip replacement. Waiting for the operation, I am told to get into the hospital gown and wait in a cubicle. Five hours later the doctor comes in with a felt tip, asks me which leg it is, draws a cross on it and leaves.'

Various obstacles to relationship are noted, including time constraints, insufficient opportunity, and perceived lack of interest. One man says: 'The young doctors, they're all too busy, they don't know what they're doing, and they don't really care.' A young man talking of his past experience with psychiatrists said that they didn't take time to listen and explore his problems, they simply made assumptions and drew up a 'map of my life in three minutes.'

How to hear what isn't said

This means being open to emotional communication. We generally hear the words and gather the facts, and we usually notice the appearance of emotions – but frequently do not pursue them.

Salinsky & Sackin (2000) reported how becoming more aware of their own feelings made doctors more aware of the feelings that their patients were experiencing and trying to communicate to them:

> *They seemed to be listening more closely without needing to interrupt the patient. There was an increase in self-reflection. While listening to the patient they were also listening to themselves. Stay with the*

pain, one doctor now says to himself. Whatever's going on, don't be deflected. Several were much more aware of their own emotional reactions to what the patient was saying.

Salinsky & Sackin (2000) conclude that 'by sharing their feelings we would become available to our patients in a way that is helpful and healing.' Listening to a person's feelings validates them and allows that person to process them. Showing compassion allows 'messy' feelings such as anger, shame and fear – which are common reactions to illness – to be accepted and integrated rather than rejected or ignored. Levenstein *et al.* (1989) state that 'patients may not necessarily articulate feelings explicitly; they are frequently under the surface, or even unconscious, often emerging during the process of the interaction.'

The patient may be grappling with a range of difficult emotions. They are trying to adjust to the reality of their illness. They are bringing to the situation emotions from their past which affect how they respond to the doctor, and how they cope with the stress of illness. The doctor responds not by reacting or withdrawing, but instead by helping the patient to stay with the feelings, and acknowledging how important they are. Bub (2006) explains that 'healing involves mourning and integrating loss. It is often a painful experience... As a result, many avoid the work of healing, and choose instead to be comforted and to move on hoping that time will heal.'

Doctors may not want to engage in this work with the patient. Zoppi & Epstein (2002) state that 'many obstacles to true caring about a patient are within the physician.' Pendleton *et al.* (2003) explain that many doctors 'develop closed and protective styles of communication.' Salinsky & Sackin (2000) state that 'doctors often develop powerful defence mechanisms to protect themselves. Some defences are essential if the doctor is to survive and to continue to function professionally. But excessive and unnecessary defences simply prevent him from listening with empathy.'

Matthews *et al.* (1993) comment that:

> *fostering greater intimacy with patients brings us more deeply into their experiences. We cannot listen empathically to their*

153

descriptions of pain without feeling it ourselves. Moreover, the issues that they bring to us often resonate with our own unresolved griefs or remind us of our own unhealed wounds. Without some source of strong grounding and support, we could easily become engulfed in or overwhelmed by the suffering we encounter and our inability to fix it.

DeLahunta & Tulsky (1996) conducted an anonymous postal survey of medical students and full-time faculty in a medical centre in New York, and found that 'a minimum of 17% of the female medical students and faculty and 3% of the male medical students and faculty have experienced physical abuse or sexual abuse by a partner in their adult life.' These figures were comparable with the general population national estimates for family violence.

A later study by Ambuel *et al.* (2003) at a medical school in the United States found that 39% of medical students reported having personally experienced severe violence in adolescence, while 19% reported forced or coerced sexual contact. They point out that 'a history of exposure to severe violence may be one factor that contributes to risk among medical students for depression, suicidal ideation and suicide.'

It is clear that patients evoke a range of difficult emotions in doctors. It appears from these studies that one of the reasons that some doctors may not wish to explore these feelings is that they touch too deeply on past personal traumatic experiences. Instead, the feelings are ignored or denied rather than acknowledging that there is personal therapeutic work to be done.

A further issue is that if doctors are not willing to engage with patients' feelings, then they may not pick up symptoms of mental illness in their patients. It has been pointed out that 'depression is among the most common conditions in primary care patients, yet studies find that physicians do not adequately detect or treat 40% to 60% of cases' (Center *et al.*, 2003).

Haidet & Paterniti (2003) encourage us towards mindful practice: 'the ability of the physician to observe not only the patient during the medical interview, but himself/herself as well.' In this way, learning about ourselves informs our interaction with others.

Salinsky & Sackin (2000) make the point that 'much of our argument is about the need for doctors to understand themselves better so that they can bring to consciousness at least some of the personal factors which prevent them from engaging in the best way with their patients.'

Therapeutic communication and intervention

Medicine is no longer simply the treatment or prevention of ill-health, it is also concerned with the definition and realisation of well-being. This is a broader issue than physical state, it also encompasses mental, emotional and spiritual state. Pendleton *et al.* (2003) state that 'spirituality generally relates to better mental health, greater well-being, and higher quality of life.' They quote Labonte (1993) who identified six components of good health:

1. Feeling vital and full of energy;
2. Having good social relationships;
3. Experiencing some control over one's life and living conditions;
4. Being able to do things one enjoys;
5. Having a sense of purpose in life;
6. Experiencing being part of a community.

In recent times a number of authors have been examining the therapeutic interaction in more depth. Teutsch (2003) states that 'sometimes the patient gains therapeutic benefit just from venting concerns in a safe environment with a caring clinician.' Tomm (1988) states that 'therapeutic conversations are organized by the desire to relieve mental pain and suffering and to produce healing.' His view is that for example, when a therapist asks questions, 'clients are stimulated to think through their problems on their own.' Questions provoke thought and emotion, but they also reveal meaning. Insights arise, and understanding grows through answering questions that have not been asked before.

Bub (2006) writes that 'healing only begins when emotions are expressed and the entire being is involved.' He explains that:

> *Healing does not occur in isolation, it emerges from a healing relationship. Communication heals when it provides safety, support,*

relief of isolation, encourages re-telling of the trauma story, reflects back the best self of the individual, reminds the patient of his/her identity besides that of patient, and supports the processing and integration of emotion.

Gilbert (2009), the originator of compassion-focused therapy, writes that: 'by demonstrating the skills and attributes of compassion – warmth, empathy, sensitivity, distress tolerance and being non-judgemental – the therapist can instil them in the client. Thus the client is helped to develop an internal compassionate relationship with themselves.'

Being authentic in the moment

- Being authentic means bringing the whole of yourself to your interactions with patients – being genuine, spontaneous, thinking and feeling. Patients can see if we are defensive, closed down, inaccessible.
- Being flexible. Be prepared to try different approaches – if one doesn't work, then try another.
- You cannot be formulaic. What works for one person will often not work for another. Each patient is different; everyone wants to feel unique, important and individual.
- Communication is about relationship – you have to connect before you can truly communicate.
- Remembering Confucius: 'Never impose on others what you would not choose for yourself.'

Chapter 9
Life and death

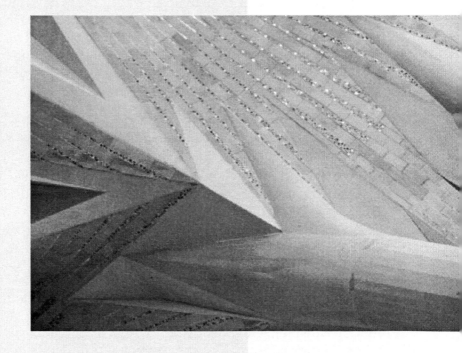

Life and death

Introduction to breaking bad news

Garg *et al.* (1997) state that 'breaking bad news is one of the most difficult tasks a physician or any other member of the health care team has to do. The way it is done may change the nature of the relationship permanently – strengthening it, undermining it, damaging it irreparably or even leading to litigation.'

Dosanjh *et al.* (2001) write that:

> *Although many health care professionals deliver 'bad news' on a daily basis, most feel uncomfortable and relatively unprepared for the interaction. In most circumstances, the delivery of bad news is a life altering experience for patients and families. Therefore, physicians at all stages of their careers should endeavour to relay 'bad news' to patients with the utmost sensitivity.*

Dosanjh *et al.* (2001) conducted a focus group to examine residents' perceptions of barriers to delivering bad news. They found that institutional barriers included lack of support and lack of available time. Personal issues were: not having time to prepare; not being able to deal with the emotional reactions and needs of patients and families; and not having the means of processing their own emotions after the delivery of bad news.

Orlander *et al.* (2002) reported that 73% of trainees first delivered bad news as a medical student or intern. For this first experience, most (61%) knew the patient for just hours or days. Only 59% engaged in any planning for the encounter. An attending physician was present in 5% of instances, and a more-senior trainee in 11%.

However, it is not only junior doctors who have difficulties. Fallowfield & Jenkins (1999) report that within oncology, 'many patients leave consultations unsure about the diagnosis and prognosis, confused about the meaning of – and need for – further diagnostic tests, unclear about the management plan and uncertain about the true therapeutic intent of treatment.' Ford *et al.* in 1996 found that dealing with patients' emotional reactions to cancer was one of the primary areas of communication difficulty for senior cancer clinicians attending training courses in England. Indeed, a survey of oncologists conducted by Baile *et al.* (1999) reported that 'cancer clinicians do not receive routine training in the psychosocial aspects of patient care such as how to communicate bad news or respond to patients who have unrealistic expectations of cure.' They found that dealing with emotion was by far the most difficult element in breaking bad news. Fallowfield & Jenkins (1999) describe insufficient training in communication and management skills as a major factor contributing to stress, lack of job satisfaction and emotional burnout in oncology.

So how do we define bad news? Ptacek & Eberhardt (1995) define it as 'situations where there is either a feeling of no hope, a threat to a person's mental or physical well being, a risk of upsetting an established lifestyle, or where a message is given which conveys to an individual fewer choices in his or her life.' The BMA (2004) quote Buckman (1984) who defines bad news as 'information likely to alter drastically a patient's view of his or her future.'

Travaline *et al.* (2005) state that 'the physician who can communicate bad news in a direct and compassionate way will not only help the patient cope, but will also strengthen the therapeutic relationship, so that it endures and further extends the healing process.'

Girgis & Sanson-Fisher (1995) outline a summary of principles for breaking bad news:

1. One person only should be responsible for breaking bad news.
2. The patient has a legal and moral right to information.
3. Primary responsibility is to the individual patient.
4. Give accurate and reliable information.
5. Ask people how much they want to know.
6. Prepare the patient for the possibility of bad news as early as possible.
7. Avoid giving the results of each test individually, if several tests are being performed.
8. Tell the patient his/her diagnosis as soon as it is certain.
9. Ensure privacy and make the patient feel comfortable.
10. Ideally, family and significant others should be present.

11. If possible, arrange for another health professional to be present.
12. Inform the patient's general practitioner and other medical advisers of level of development of patient's understanding.
13. Use eye contact and body language to convey warmth, sympathy, encouragement, or reassurance to the patient.
14. Employ a trained health interpreter if language differences exist.
15. Be sensitive to the person's culture, race, religious beliefs, and social background.
16. Acknowledge your own shortcomings and emotional difficulties in breaking bad news.

Travaline *et al.* (2005) detail a list of practical steps:

1. Assess what the patient already knows about his or her condition to prevent confusion when new information is introduced.
2. Assess what the patient wants to know: not all patients with the same diagnosis want the same level of detail in the information offered about their condition or treatment.
3. Be empathic: recognize, acknowledge and explore the indirectly expressed emotions of patients.
4. Slow down: provide information in a slow and deliberate fashion, pause frequently.
5. Keep it simple: short statements and clear, simple explanations.
6. Tell the truth.
7. Be hopeful: being able to promise comfort and minimal suffering has real value.
8. Watch the patient's body and face: facial expressions are often good indicators of sadness, worry, or anxiety.
9. Be prepared for a reaction: give sufficient time for a full display of emotions, listen quietly and attentively to what the patient or family are saying.

How to break bad news

Bad news is likely to be unwelcome, shocking, and life-changing. As a doctor, you cannot change the fact that bad news is bad. Once said, it cannot be taken back. Some people may have been expecting the news, for others it may come as a total surprise – either way, it is important to allow patients and relatives time and space to feel their emotions.

There are many different types of bad news. As a doctor, you cannot necessarily tell what will or will not be bad news. Giving a diagnosis, talking about the meaning of symptoms, telling a patient that they will lose a limb, or lose the ability to move or to function in some way, or discussing disease progression can all be extremely upsetting and difficult for patients to hear. In addition to the possibility of loss of life itself, there is loss of the way of life, changes that mean that a person is no longer independent, able to manage their own affairs, able to do the things they love to do. You cannot make any assumptions about how an individual will react to any particular piece of news, or which aspects will be most distressing or difficult for them to come to terms with.

Assessment of urgency

The first thing to decide is the degree of urgency in telling the bad news. This depends firstly on the patient's clinical condition, for example, if a patient has developed a spinal cord compression, you will have to tell them quickly in order to organise urgent treatment. In other circumstances, for example if the patient has established disease such as cancer, and test results have come back showing disease progression, then you will need time to discuss this fully. If you are rushed or under pressure, then it is better to postpone it and come back later when you may have more time. If the patient is pressurising you for news of the results, then you may need to tell them as soon as you have the results.

Breaking bad news doesn't have to be done all in one session. It can be a process over time.

Self-preparation

In preparing for the discussion, make sure you have all the facts before giving the news. Look at the scans, read the notes and reports, and have it clear in your mind, then you can go through it logically with the patient. If despite this, you can't remember some details during the conversation, then you can be honest and say 'I can't remember,' or 'I don't know, but I will find out and come back to you on that.' Reading the notes may also give you some indication as to what has been said so far.

Before going to see the patient or relatives, it is a good idea to give yourself time to calm yourself, and to think about how you are going to start the conversation. It may be helpful to talk it through with someone else, for example another member of the team who knows the patient or has met the family. Then, find a quiet place for a few minutes before going to talk to the patient. Be aware of your own feelings for the person – it may be upsetting if you like the person or have become fond of them. On the other hand, it may be harder to deal with people who have been angry and difficult on the ward, with patients or relatives who have complained about something, or those who have unrealistic expectations.

In practice, junior doctors see patients most frequently, and they have less experience and knowledge than their senior colleagues, which can make it difficult to answer patients' questions. For example, a junior doctor told a woman with melanoma while her sons were present that the ultrasound scan of her liver had shown that she had metastases. Unfortunately the doctor had not found out prior to the conversation what would happen next as a result of this finding. The doctor was honest about not knowing and offered to speak with her seniors and return as soon as possible. This was a reasonable thing to do but it would perhaps have been better to have found this out beforehand.

Practical issues

Find the right place to give the news. It needs to be private and you need to have enough time to talk it through. Every situation is different. Some people just want the straight facts, not the explanations, and others may need longer to ask questions or just to take it all in. This means the amount of time needed can be extremely variable. Doctors on hospital wards may find it very difficult to find adequate space and time. On one occasion I had to talk to a patient and his relatives in the corridor. I found a cubby hole and put some chairs in there. There was no alternative, but it really was unacceptable. Sometimes there is no alternative but to give the news at the bedside if the patient is unable to get out of bed to go to a private room.

Try not to inadvertently tell the patient the bad news before you get there. A consultant arranged a meeting with a patient to break the bad news that he had lung cancer. His wife had been contacted and she was in the room with her husband. The nurses had made them both a pot of tea. As soon as the consultant entered the room the man said: 'I know what you're going to tell me because the best china's out!'

It is good practice to try and get rid of your bleep and phone for the duration of the interview. It is best to write in the notes after the conversation. Having a colleague sit in the corner writing during the conversation can be perceived as insensitive.

I encourage junior doctors to sit in a few times with me before they give bad news alone.

Determining what patients know already and how much information they want

When you first meet a patient it's a good idea to take the opportunity to ask what the patient already knows about their illness. It's also a good idea at an early stage to ask people how much information they want, especially if you know that there will be a specific conversation that you're going to have to have with them at some point. For example you may have ordered a CT scan to assess their response to chemotherapy. I might say: 'Are you the sort of person who needs to know everything? Everyone's different, and some people want to know all the facts, and others are happy to leave decisions to doctors. What sort of person are you with regards to this?' It can be comforting to know the answer to this question, as then you will later know that you're doing it right for that person.

A lot of the time a person will tell you clearly what they have been told so far which is extremely helpful. On occasions people might say 'I don't know anything.' Perhaps they really haven't been told much previously, perhaps they haven't been able to take it all in – occasionally it might be denial. When patients say: 'The doctors haven't told me anything,' it may be that they have had a bad communication experience, therefore they are more closed and defensive, which makes things more difficult. The important thing is to show that person that you're there to help, that you have time to spend with them and that you are happy to go over anything they need to talk about. Being kind and showing the patient that you do want to talk about what's important for them will help to repair the situation. If someone says they haven't been told anything try to gently explore it a bit further. Ask the question slightly differently for example: 'Do you recall what the tests have shown so far?'

Determining whether to tell a patient alone or with relatives

It's a good idea to ask the patient at the first meeting or when clerking them onto the ward who they agree for you to share information with. Ask: 'Are you happy for me to talk to your relatives, and is there anyone you do not wish me to share information with?'

In some settings such as a hospice, you may see people and their relatives on the ward over a number of days, and there is often opportunity to talk regularly. You can then get to know them and it's easier to judge whether the patient would like the relatives to be there when you tell them bad news. If you do not know the patient, then you can start to get to know them and build up some rapport so that it is easier to judge whether they would need a relative with them when you give them bad news. You may ask, 'Do you want your relatives to be there for the results of the scan?' It may be that a family comes in to talk about the results, and hordes of people arrive all at once. In this case it can be very stressful to deal with so many people. It is reasonable to ask to speak to just one or two. It is appropriate to ask the patient who they would like to be there or which of their relatives would be best to speak to.

It is not good practice to speak to relatives before the patient. Some relatives ask you to collude with them regarding the patient's illness. They might ask you about the diagnosis when the patient is out of the room, or might say, 'Don't tell them, they couldn't cope with knowing.' This is a very difficult situation. The family are obviously trying to protect someone they love from being hurt and upset. This needs to be acknowledged. It needs to be explained that the person will have picked up on nonverbal clues and they may be confused by not having a reason for their ongoing symptoms and this might be more frightening for them. Also explain to them in the case of a progressive illness such as cancer that it will be harder to conceal the diagnosis as time goes on. Explain that you need to offer the patient the opportunity to talk about what is happening and to discuss any test results. Explain that you will do this sensitively, and would not force any information upon them.

Giving the news

There are a few golden rules in giving news: don't lie, don't use jargon, don't use euphemisms and listen to the patient.

People's intuition is frequently accurate. Often they know what is happening to their body and have a good idea of what that means. Sometimes doctors do not take patients' fears or opinions seriously enough. For example, one conversation went badly from the start:

> **Patient:** 'I think that since my last visit, the cancer has started to spread, because there seem to be some more lumps on the other side of my neck.'

> **Doctor (not her usual consultant) [examines her]:** 'I think you're getting paranoid. There really is no evidence of your cancer spreading. You need to get a grip on yourself and not let your imagination run away with you.'

> (The following week, the patient's own consultant confirmed a spread of the disease, which meant that the course of treatment had to be altered).

It is a good idea to give a 'warning shot' when breaking bad news, for example 'I have come to talk to you about the results of your tests and I'm afraid it's not what we had hoped for.' In the case of a diagnosis of cancer, you may use words such as 'growth' or 'tumour' but it is very important to actually use the word 'cancer' at some point. In the case of speaking to a family you may begin by saying something like: 'It seems your mother's condition has changed over the past few days,' or 'It seems she has deteriorated.' At some point it may be important to use the word 'dying.'

When I was a houseman on a respiratory ward, one of the doctors did a bronchoscopy list one day and would then tell the patients the following morning what had been found. On one occasion, a woman and her daughter were waiting to go home, and the doctor came in and said, 'We looked down and there was a swelling.' He repeated the word 'swelling' several times, and they left. On their way out, I heard them saying, 'Thank God, it's just a swelling.'

It is important to explain things in a clear, understandable way. Avoid jargon. It is so easy to use medical terms without thinking. Wherever possible try to check back with the person to make sure they have understood what has been said so far.

The conversation does not end after the news has been broken. Although you have achieved what you needed to, it is the patient's agenda you should be following. The important thing is to have a conversation. Show empathy, allow silences. It is often true that the longer the silence, the more important the next bit of information. Emotional work is being done. If the silence becomes uncomfortable, don't break it, feel yourself becoming uncomfortable and allow it to continue. Reflecting back what someone has said to you shows empathy, for example if someone says: 'This is absolutely awful,' I might say: 'Yes, it is awful.'

Body language conveys a lot of information. If you genuinely feel concern then this will be reflected in both your verbal and nonverbal communication. If you are having to think about your body language, then it's likely that it won't be natural and won't come across as such. Touching a person who is upset may be comforting and show warmth and sympathy, maybe just a touch on their arm. It's best to go with what feels natural, your intuitive sense of whether it is appropriate or not will guide you. Some people will put their hand above the patient's hand so that the patient can easily move if they feel uncomfortable.

Give the patient time to take in the news you have just given them.

It is likely that questions will follow. Questions clarifying what you have said, questions about treatment, questions about the future. Some questions are easier to answer, for example what further investigations are necessary, or what treatment the patient is going to receive. Others are more difficult; you cannot give a precise time scale, and you can't predict exactly what the effects or side-effects of treatment will be. It is important to be honest about that, and to communicate any uncertainty to the patient. Many doctors find uncertainty threatening, they may find it difficult, or they may feel personally inadequate to admit that they don't know.

Discussing the prognosis

After conversations such as giving the diagnosis of cancer or telling a relative that their loved one is now dying you will often be asked about prognosis. Always make sure you are answering the right question. 'How long have I got?' might mean 'How long have I got until I go home?' Once you have established that the person has asked how long they have left to live, ask whether this is something they really want answered now. It may be that they feel this is what they should be asking but actually are not quite ready to hear the answer. You can never give a precise answer and you need to be honest about this. It can be important to a person to know an estimate in order to prepare both practically and emotionally. The time scale is determined by the rate of change of disease or symptoms for that individual, there is no definitive answer. It can be helpful to say: 'It seems that things have been changing over the past few weeks. We need to be guided by that.' It is best to say in terms of 'days,' 'weeks to months' or 'months' depending on the rate of change. Using specific numbers of months such as 'six to nine months' can be unhelpful. If a person dies before six months, the family may feel cheated, and if they live beyond nine months this conversation can still be hanging over them.

It is always very difficult to try to predict how long a person has to live. Never guess, and always ask colleagues, either for their opinion or for them to have the discussion themselves if you don't feel confident. Sometimes it is just impossible to even estimate and although the uncertainty can be very hard for the patient or relative, honesty is important.

People react to the answers to this question very differently and no assumptions can be made. There may be fear about dying. If someone expresses such a fear it may be appropriate to explore further. Many people are frightened about the process of dying itself, worried that they might be sick or that the pain might get worse, in which case you can reassure a lot by telling them that you will take care to control their pain or other symptoms. Some people are afraid of what might happen to them after death. It can be helpful to help them to distinguish between the two issues. A person may find it useful to talk to a priest or chaplain.

Allowing the patient to react

When giving bad news, the results of tests or a diagnosis, it may come as a complete surprise to the patient, and they will need time to react. A person may be acutely distressed, upset or angry, or numb from shock and completely unable to take in what has been said. One woman described the following conversation:

> Consultant: 'I'm afraid the biopsy shows that you have Hodgkin's disease.'
>
> Patient: 'What's that?'
>
> Consultant: 'Lymph cancer.'
>
> Patient: [starts to cry]
>
> Consultant: 'Don't cry – by next time I see you, you will feel really silly about having got upset like this today.'
>
> Patient: [having composed herself] 'Can it be treated?'
>
> Consultant: 'Yes, it is one of the easier cancers to treat. If I had to choose one to have, I would most definitely choose that one...or maybe testicular cancer... but I think you would have difficulty getting that one!'

It helps to see people as people and not just patients. Different people react in different ways to bad news. Don't assume that because people are young that it will be harder or that if they are old it will be easier to hear that they have a terminal illness or are dying. In fact, it's best not to assume anything, but to ask questions and find out how they are feeling about what you have said.

Remember that bad news is bad news and you can't change that, but how the patient or their relatives react is partially dependent on how you've done the talking so far. You know fairly soon after meeting people how well you connect, and you then build the relationship in a stepwise manner, building rapport and trust as things unfold. Be sensitive to their responses. As they react in a certain way, you allow them to be what they need to be at that time, and support them. Allow them to express themselves in whatever way they need to, and acknowledge it, 'It's ok,' let them cry, don't try to stop them. This process cannot be formulaic; you have to be closely in touch with your own sensitivity and intuition.

People can respond to bad news with anger, or by blaming other people: 'Why did the GP miss this?' 'Why wasn't it found sooner?' Let people get it off their chest, and acknowledge their feelings. On occasions people can be so angry about a previous issue that they are unable to address what is happening currently. You need to bring them back to the focus of the here and now especially if someone is dying and time is short. Acknowledge how they are feeling, advise them to address it in some way in the future but to put it to one side for now.

If people are angry, don't get angry yourself, because in the main it is not related to you, but recognise that they may be angry with you for delivering the message, in which case you do have to just take it on the chin a bit. Rarely, someone is so angry that you just have to close the session and return later.

Sometimes people find it too upsetting to talk at all about any of the details of their illness. Offer the opportunity to talk about things later: 'There may be things you want to talk about or ask about later and we're willing to talk about those at any time.' Don't close the door on them just because they're not ready to discuss things at that point. People differ in how they process emotions and how they deal with difficulties. Listen and empathise.

Hope and support

If there is no further active treatment that will be helpful, or no hope of cure, it's important to explain what happens next. 'We will continue to support you. We will control your symptoms as much as we can.' Then there is still some hope.

Sometimes, however, there is nothing you can say. When you can't help someone, what do you do? Just being there helps. That's part of our role as doctors – 'cure sometimes, relieve often, be there always.'

It is also important to allow yourself to feel your own emotions, your eyes may fill up, or you may want to go off to a quiet place for ten minutes afterwards to centre yourself and feel balanced again.

Offering time to answer questions and to talk

Ask the patient or relative whether they have any questions and reassure them that they can come back in the future if they think of things that they would like to ask. 'I'm here all afternoon,' or 'I will be here tomorrow, let the nurses know that you want to talk to me and I'm happy to come back.' People take time to assimilate information and to process emotions, therefore there may be a need for further discussion when they are ready. People may need to hear things several times in order to be able to take in all the details.

A person may want you to be present when they tell relatives the news. If they need to tell children, then it is particularly helpful to involve a health professional such as a social worker who has experience in dealing with children.

Communication and documentation

It can be helpful to take someone in with you when you have to break bad news, for example an experienced nurse, health care assistant, or another doctor. It is also very important to communicate with other members of the team immediately after breaking bad news – talk to the nurses straight afterwards, hand over what you have said, and write it in the notes so that the whole team know how the patient will be affected by what they know.

You must also write in the medical notes which relatives the patient wants you to share information with, and the names of any who they do not wish to tell. It is important to contact the GP as family members may go to them for support.

The dying patient

When talking to family members about a relative who is dying, it is helpful to prepare them as much as possible for the changes they might see in the patient, such as becoming more sleepy, eating and drinking less. Reassure them that changes in breathing such as noises due to secretions are unlikely to be distressing to the patient. As relatives may be with the person for a great deal of the time at this stage, ask them to call the nurse should they be worried about the person's comfort in any way.

Coping with dying and looking after yourself

Your past experiences affect how you feel about death and dying. Your attitudes and beliefs affect your actions. It is important to talk to someone about your feelings. Some palliative care teams have a psychologist who supports the team. There may be a reflective practice group, which can be a helpful forum in which to discuss particularly distressing cases. However, in practice there is often no protected time or no one to facilitate the group. Within the team, then, you may be able to share the load, perhaps by taking it in turns to see the most upsetting patients. Talking to colleagues, friends, or partners is a common way of processing some of the feelings that arise during the course of work. A 'difficult case' session facilitated by a psychologist can be helpful, whether run from an analytical or supportive standpoint. Balint groups may also be helpful. In any event, self-reflection is vital, asking yourself about why you felt as you did in a particular situation and giving yourself time to reflect on how your own experiences have shaped your reactions to others.

If a person has had upsetting experiences and has not dealt with their feelings, then these may interfere with the ability to support the patient and relatives through their own emotional process of adaptation and grieving. For example, a situation arose when a patient under the care of the palliative care team was admitted to hospital acutely unwell with a potentially reversible problem. He had a reasonable prognosis with regard to his cancer, and difficult decisions needed to be made with regard to various treatment options. A member of staff involved in the man's care became quite angry during these discussions, making comments about his own experience of his father's death from cancer in an acute hospital, which he had obviously found very distressing.

The process of breaking bad news and caring for people as they adjust to that news can be very rewarding. Surprisingly, people say 'Thank you' at the end of that discussion. It is a hugely important event for that person, and it's vital to take the time to learn how to do it well. They are likely to remember it forever.

Supporting relatives through their grief is also a hugely important task, and one that doctors in general practice and all specialities will be faced with at some point in time. One relative writes:

> *My dad was becoming more and more breathless. He had lung cancer, and the doctors had told us he had only months to live. That night he was lying on the sofa, and his breathing started to get even worse. He usually felt better when he was sitting up, so I went over and lifted him up in my arms. I said to mum to phone the doctor. His breathing sounded very strange, and then it just stopped and he died in my arms. I still remember how shocked I was that he had actually died. I was appalled by the fact that there was nothing I could do to save him. I ran up to my room and started crying uncontrollably. I heard the doctor arrive, but he didn't come up to see me. My mum didn't either. Later, my mum said that the doctor had told her just to leave me alone in my room. I was a medical student at the time.*

End-of-life care

In the United Kingdom almost a quarter of occupied hospital bed days are taken up by patients who are in the last year of life, and some 60% of all deaths occur there (Clark, 2005).

The term 'palliative care' was first proposed in 1974 by the Canadian surgeon, Balfour Mount (Clark, 2005). The World Health Organisation (WHO) defines it as 'the active total care of patients whose disease is not responsive to curative treatment. Control of pain, of other symptoms and of psychological, social and spiritual problems is paramount. The goal of palliative care is achievement of the best possible quality of life for patients and their families' (Saunders, 1996).

Dame Cicely Saunders, who founded the first hospice in the UK, St Christopher's Hospice in Sydenham, in 1967, wrote in 1958: 'It seems to me that many patients feel deserted by their doctors at the end. Ideally the doctor should remain the centre of a team who work together to relieve where they cannot heal, to keep the patient's own struggle within his compass and to bring hope and consolation to the end' (Clark, 2005).

Saunders revolutionised the care of the dying. Her view was that 'constant pain needs constant control,' and she described the concept of 'total pain, which was presented as a complex of physical, emotional, social, and spiritual elements. The whole experience for a patient includes anxiety, depression, and fear; concern for the family who will become bereaved; and often a need to find some meaning in the situation, some deeper reality in which to trust' (Saunders, 1996).

'Kubler-Ross (1970) writes of the changing expressions of grief which should be taken into account: despair, denial, anger, bargaining, depression and acceptance, not necessarily always in that order' (RCP, 1997).

It is important that the doctor finds himself able to talk about these issues and to deal with the emotions that inevitably accompany them. Sensitive communication and the ability to support the patient may at some point become more valuable than medical treatments and interventions. Indeed, Buckman (2002) makes the point that 'communication is often a major component of the medical management in chronic and palliative care: sometimes it is all we have to offer.'

Ptacek & Eberhardt (1996) reported that when they were being given bad news, 'patients wanted their physician to be honest, compassionate and caring, hopeful, and informative. They wanted to be told in person, in a private setting, at their own pace with time for discussion, and with a supportive person present.' They found that the majority of patients were satisfied with the way it had been done, although some wanted more information, more opportunity to show their feelings, or more emotional support from the doctor delivering the news.

Clark (2005) quotes Saunders (1963) who wrote that:

> *Mental distress may be perhaps the most intractable pain of all for which listening has to develop into real hearing. Indeed, physical and mental suffering are seen almost dialectically: each capable of influencing and shaping the other. If physical symptoms are alleviated then mental pain is lifted also.*

Recent research has shown that uneasiness with death and dying is of concern for many doctors, maybe because they feel ineffective and powerless (Dosanjh *et al.*, 2001) and therefore 'limit their relationship with the patient or the patient's family members to areas where they feel comfortable' (Girgis & Sanson-Fisher, 1995), or because they fear that 'if they clarified how a dying patient was feeling they could unleash strong emotions like despair and anger that they could not contain' (Maguire, 1985).

The Royal College of Physicians (1997) state that:

> *Doctors become anxious about giving bad news because they fear that patients will become distressed, emotionally disorganised, ask difficult or impossible questions, express disappointment, blame or anger and will find it unusually difficult to see the clinical facts in perspective. Doctors also fear being in a position of not knowing all the answers, the loss of the familiar support of clinical authority and loss of control. They may also be aware that they do not have the skill to comfort distressed patients and relatives and also that to do so threatens to be time-consuming.*

Maguire (1985) reports that:

> *direct observation of doctors and nurses talking with real, simulated, or role played patients suffering from a terminal illness has shown that they consistently use distancing tactics. These prevent them getting close to their patients' psychological suffering and are used to try to ensure their own emotional survival. Since these tactics discourage patients from disclosing their psychological concerns they are a serious barrier to effective psychological care.*

Doctors are often unaware that they are using these distancing tactics, which include: the use of false reassurance, making more positive statements than are warranted, and selective attention; following up only physical symptoms when a patient complains of both physical and psychological difficulties (Maguire, 1985). The use of leading questions, focusing on and clarifying physical aspects, and moving into advice and reassurance mode have all been found to inhibit patient disclosure (Maguire *et al.*, 1996b).

Yet it is known that psychological morbidity in patients with cancer is high. Fallowfield *et al.* (1990) found that in women with a diagnosis of breast cancer, rates of anxiety, depression, and sexual dysfunction were high, both in those undergoing mastectomy and lumpectomy. 21% of women who underwent mastectomy were depressed.

Maguire (2000) reports that:

> *patients who have undergone major surgery, such as the removal of a breast, say it is rare for them to be asked by anyone involved in their care how they felt about the surgery and how they have reacted to it. In the absence of such explicit enquiry, they believe that doctors are not interested in learning about the effect of the surgery on them. Therefore they feel that it is not legitimate to mention any problems spontaneously.*

Newell *et al.* (1998) quote studies suggesting that:

> *up to 91% of patients who receive chemotherapy experience elevated levels of anxiety and up to 61% experience depression (Nerenz et al., 1982; Jacobsen et al., 1993; Carroll et al., 1993). Furthermore, many aspects of patients' quality of life are also diminished: their physical and work activities are reduced, their social activities are disrupted, family and other relationships often deteriorate, their level of sexual activity decreases, and they often find themselves under increasing financial burdens (Gilbar, 1991; Meyerowitz et al., 1983).*

If psychological issues are not explored, important problems can be overlooked. Newell *et al.* (1998) report that only 17% of patients classified as clinically anxious and 6% of those classified as clinically depressed were perceived as such by their oncologists.

Maguire (1985) makes the point that 'doctors and nurses assume that patients who develop psychological problems will disclose them. So they rarely inquire directly about how dying patients are adjusting emotionally. They are also uncertain about how to distinguish between worry and an anxiety state and between sadness and a depressive illness.'

However, MacDonald (2004) states that 'allowing patients to talk about their predicament and concerns, providing they wish to, is perceived by patients and carers as therapeutic and usually eases the emotional burden they experience.' The point is that doctors don't need to provide the answers all the time, they just need to listen. Giving people time and space to express their feelings, and being concerned for them, allows them an opportunity to feel supported within what is actually a very powerful relationship. The last thing the patient wants is to feel rejected by their doctor. Healing occurs through giving time, learning to speak about things without your own feelings getting in the way, and, in the end, just being there.

Chapter 10

Dealing with difficult situations

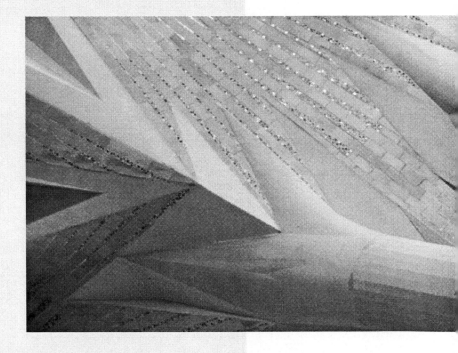

Dealing with difficult situations

Managing conflict in the team

In their report on medical professionalism, the Royal College of Physicians (2005) stated that:

> *The keys to strong clinical teams are recognition, mutual respect, and an appreciation of the constant redefinition of boundaries among the team. Overall, doctors have not spent sufficient time learning from other members of the healthcare team (e.g. ward-based patient handovers by nurses). The truth is that, in practice, doctors have insufficient time for effective team-building. They are often confused about their roles. And the vertical management of separate professional groupings tends to undermine the goals and work of a cross-disciplinary team.*

Coombs (2003) states that 'current government policy places increasing emphasis on the need for flexible team working. This requires a shared understanding of roles and working practices. However, review of the current literature reveals that such a collaborative working environment has not as yet, been fully achieved.'

For example, Coombs & Ersser (2004) report that there has been much debate on the nature of working relationships within the health care team. In a study examining clinical decision-making in intensive care units, they found that 'conflict arose between doctors and nurses, in particular because medicine dominated the decision-making process. The nursing role, whilst pivotal to implementing clinical decisions, remained unacknowledged and devalued. Medical hegemony continues to render nurses unable to influence substantially the decision-making process.'

Willard & Luker (2007) state that in the recent reorganisation of cancer services in the UK, the nurse specialist was given a new and different role as a core member of the multiprofessional team. However, they found that 'acceptance, especially by doctors, was the main problem facing cancer nurse specialists. In addition, they experienced insufficient organizational support for their role. Difficulties with acceptance impaired nurses' ability to provide supportive care to cancer patients. Nurse specialists responded by employing several strategies including building relationships and establishing role boundaries.'

Coombs (2003) report that 'role definitions and power bases based on traditional and historical boundaries continue to exist.' For example, in their study in intensive care, they found that 'whilst the nursing role in intensive care has changed, this has had little impact on how clinical decisions are made. Both medical and nursing staff identify conflict during patient management discussions.'

Rafferty *et al.* (2001) conducted a postal survey of 10,022 staff nurses in 32 hospitals in England to explore the relationship between interdisciplinary teamwork and nurse autonomy. They found that 'nurses with higher teamwork scores also exhibited higher levels of autonomy and were more involved in decision-making. A strong association was found between teamwork and autonomy; this interaction suggests synergy rather than conflict. Organisations should therefore be encouraged to promote nurse autonomy without fearing that it might undermine teamwork.'

Castledine (2008) state that:

> *dealing with difficult doctors is not easy, and often many nurses shrink away from conflict situations because they are too intimidated to fight back. Unfortunately, despite years of study and comment, there is still a feeling that some doctors regard nurses as their hand-maidens. To explain this attitude as just a battle of feminine and masculine identity would be very short-sighted as studies have suggested that there is more to the nurse/doctor relationship than following a medical model of treatment.*

The RCP report (2005) states that:

> *there is relatively little knowledge about how teams of health professionals operate in practice. What evidence there is suggests that teams are not even close to fulfilling their real potential. Ethnographic research in hospital settings, for example, shows that collaboration between professional groups is usually short-lived, unstructured, opportunistic, fragmented, and rushed.*

'Teams in many healthcare settings, notably acute care, are inherently unstable. They are provisional, forever changing, forming and reforming with every new shift' (RCP, 2005).

With the recent introduction of the European Working Time Directive, 'the increasing use of shift systems for junior doctors can lead to a further splintering of care, making the introduction of safe methods of communication at hand-over times essential' (RCP, 1997). Murray *et al.* (2005) found that 'more than three quarters of medical senior house officers and nearly half of specialist registrars in NHS trusts were working seven consecutive night shifts when surveyed in December 2004 by the Royal College of Physicians. Thus, many of these doctors were forced to work up to 91 hours during the night in one week, as well as travelling to and from home each day.' They point out that these doctors are exhausted, leading to an increased frequency of accidents and mistakes.

In addition to safety issues, however, constant tiredness must have a negative effect on interpersonal relationships, communication, and decision-making. Tired, irritable, and overstretched, these doctors are likely to be less empathic and to have slow or impaired decision-making skills.

Awareness of the issues is the first step towards resolving some of the problems. The Medical Leadership Competency Framework drawn up by the Academy of Medical Royal Colleges and the Institute for Innovation and Improvement (2005) states that in order to be able to work within teams, doctors must:

- Have a clear sense of their role, responsibilities and purpose within the team.
- Adopt a team approach, acknowledging and appreciating efforts, contributions and compromises.
- Recognise the common purpose of the team and respect team decisions.
- Listen to others.
- Empathise and take into account the needs and feelings of others.
- Communicate effectively with individuals and groups.
- Gain and maintain the trust and support of colleagues.

The Framework states that in working with others, doctors should:

- Provide encouragement and opportunity for people to engage in decision-making.
- Respect, value and acknowledge the roles, contributions and expertise of others.
- Employ strategies to manage conflict of interests and differences of opinion.
- Keep the focus of contribution on delivering and improving services to patients.

Handling difficult patients

Maguire (2000) suggests guidelines for interviewing in difficult circumstances:

> *Ideally you should assess any new patient, whether they are acutely ill or not, in private. When you have to interview patients in restricted environments you need to be aware that they may withhold important information because they fear it will be overheard by other people. Therefore you must check later whether anything was missed out from the initial history.*

Sometimes relatives are keen to talk to the doctor before the patient has been seen. It is good practice to assess the patient first, and then to offer some time to the relatives. The patient's autonomy must be respected, and confidentiality maintained. There are occasions when patients do not want relatives to know details of their condition, and you must check first with the patient who they want information to be shared with. You cannot make assumptions about this, but must ask the patient and document it in the notes. Maguire (2000) states that 'it is best if you negotiate that it would be more helpful to see the patient alone first and then, provided that the patient agrees, you can see the relative either separately or with the patient. Most relatives accept this arrangement as they know they will have access to the doctor soon.'

However, it is sometimes not easy to discover the patient's wishes:

A patient admitted following self harm was waiting for a psychiatric assessment. A nurse had taken a phone call from his daughter who said she was on her way to the hospital, and the nurse told him this. When I arrived to assess this man, he was intensely angry. He would not engage in eye contact, was staring into space, and answered questions with the minimum information. His face was bright red with anger, and he was unable to say anything other than that he wanted me to leave him alone and we should mind our own business. I said to him, 'I'm sorry that you're so upset, and I've heard some of what's been going on for you, but I don't know the whole story. It would help me if you could explain what's been happening.'

'I'm not telling you anything.'

'I only want you to tell me what you're comfortable with. There may be things that you don't want to talk about, and that's fine.'

[Staring, silent.]

'Can you say anything about what you're feeling? I can see that things are very difficult for you at the moment.'

'This is pointless.'

'Why pointless?'

'You can't possibly understand. You think you know but you don't.'

For about fifteen minutes his hostility continued, then finally his anger broke and he told his story, that his was estranged from his family and that he did not want any information disclosed to them.

I reassured him that his wishes would be respected and we finished the assessment.

Certain patients are difficult. Serour *et al.* (2009) state that 'all physicians must care for some patients who are perceived as difficult because of behavioural or emotional aspects that affect their care.' They conducted a study of doctors working in primary care services. The majority of doctors agreed that patient characteristics that render them difficult included: psychological disorders, life stresses, social isolation, multiple physical problems, chronic diseases, inability to communicate own needs, unrealistic expectations.

However, the study found that 'the problems do not lie exclusively with the patients.' Most doctors felt that their own reasons for perceiving patients as difficult were: workload, lack of job satisfaction, their own psychic condition, and lack of training in counselling and communication skills.

Levinson *et al.* (1993) found that of doctors in busy practice settings, '36% reported frustration in 11-25% of visits. 8% felt frustrated in up to half of their patient encounters. The cause of the frustrating visits was most frequently attributed to the nature of the patient (50%).'

Smith (1995) states that 'dealing with difficult patients can represent a significant burden in the life of doctors. It is more productive, however, to view this burden as a product of the interaction between doctor and patient, for which both have a responsibility, rather than attributing any problems encountered to shortcomings of the patient alone.' For example, Rosendal *et al.* (2005) report that 'somatising patients frequently present in primary care but GPs often express frustration in dealing with them. A negative attitude may result in missed diagnoses and ineffective treatment.' Pendleton *et al.* (2003) quote Schwenk (1987) who demonstrated that difficult doctor-patient relationships were associated with two to three times higher rates of investigations and referrals.

The RCP report (1997) states that:

> *even the most devoted and concerned doctor may find that some patients are simply awkward. These patients may sometimes be untreatable in that they attend frequently, continue to complain in the face of apparently adequate conventional treatment both for physical and mental conditions, produce multiple complaints, often serially, and generally express dissatisfaction with all efforts.*

Salinsky & Sackin (2000) report that 'patients who presented themselves as emergencies were likely to incur the doctor's anger if there was no blood to be seen. Patients with strongly held health beliefs which the doctor considered absurd and unscientific could also arouse a doctor's anger.' The RCP report (1997) mentions other reasons why some patients become unpopular with their doctors: 'those who are perceived to perpetuate their problems because they do not accept medical advice or perhaps because they do not conform to the doctor's perceptions of "moral fibre." Yet others seem almost impossible to treat despite having important and potentially damaging problems, such as gross resistant obesity.' The report, while admitting that no panacea is available to help doctors deal with such patients, suggests that 'careful and repeated explanation which brings the patient and the doctor to a common understanding of a management plan, however difficult or hopeless it may be perceived to be, is as important with these patients as with others.'

If doctors do not acknowledge their frustrations and personal emotional reactions to difficult patients, then these may compound the problem. Levinson *et al.* (1993) state that:

> *physicians may unconsciously or consciously punish, confront, or try to 'get rid of' the patient. A particular physician may be upset or irritated by a patient for reasons related to the physician's own psychological or social situation. Feelings can include sadness, being overwhelmed, anger, and rejection. Finally, some physicians experience frustration in specific problem areas including alcohol, drugs, chronic pain, or somatisation.*

They suggest that doctors 'analyse the source of their frustration and seek ways to modify the experience' (Levinson *et al.*, 1993). This might involve seeking help or support from colleagues, or attending training and gaining further skills.

O'Dowd (1988) conducted a study in general practice in which heartsink patients were discussed in order to 'share information, define apparent problems, formulate a plan of management, and provide support for the professional who was to deal most with a particular patient.' Butler *et al.* (1999) suggest ways to manage the heartsink patient, including:

- Improving clinicians' self-awareness, counselling, and consultation skills.
- The doctor provides the patient with the opportunity to communicate, which can result in brief, intense, and close contact that can be deeply therapeutic.
- The 'holding strategy' whereby positive attempts to bring about change are abandoned in favour of simply listening to the patient without contradicting him/her.
- Improving doctors' working conditions to reduce stress and enable them to cope better with difficult situations.
- Enhancing understanding and sharing responsibility through team discussion.

Demanding patients or relatives

Sometimes patients or relatives can have a fixed idea of what the patient needs and what they expect from the doctor. It can be helpful early on to ask about their view of the problem, and what they were expecting in terms of treatment, so that the doctor can negotiate a shared understanding. A patient may disagree with the diagnosis, in which case it may be helpful to go through a list of diagnostic criteria with the patient to see if they feel that their symptoms fit the diagnosis that you have in mind. For instance, with patients with borderline personality disorder, it is very useful to ask the patient about each symptom and to write down the patient's answers against the list of DSM-IV (1994) criteria. You can then discuss the diagnosis together. Frequently, such patients have attracted a variety of diagnoses beforehand, such as bipolar disorder, psychosis, ADHD, or recurrent depression. However, to make a definitive diagnosis of borderline personality disorder, if this exists, is often a relief to the patient, who may never have really felt that the previous diagnoses fitted their illness pattern. It also means that they can get the most effective treatment.

On other occasions it is the treatment and management plan rather than the diagnosis that is brought into question. Levinson *et al.* (1993) state that 'demanding' patients may pressure doctors to order specific tests or insist on referrals to various specialists.' Maguire (2000) explains that:

> *Some relatives are very demanding in terms of what they expect to be done for the patient, the level of care given, investigations*

performed and treatments provided. It is important that the relatives are confronted constructively with regard to what can reasonably be done and what is unreasonable. If their demands continue, it is important to confront them with the fact that their requests are unusual, and the basis of this should be explored. This will normally be due to major fears or guilt, or anxiety that the patient might die.

Managing aggression and violence

Perrin (1997) reports that 'it has been estimated that 50% of health care staff will be physically assaulted at least once at some point in their careers.' Davies (2001) conducted a postal questionnaire of 139 doctors working in South Wales, and found that over the previous year:

> *17% of respondents reported one or more assaults, and 32% reported one or more threats. The most junior senior house officers (SHOs) were significantly more likely to have experienced an incident. Most assaults (61%) were committed by patients from general adult psychiatry, and half occurred during urgent assessments. 58% of the assailants were known to have previously assaulted a member of staff, and this information was known to the doctor before the assault for 88%. 16% of the assailants had been drinking alcohol prior to the assault.*

Forster *et al.* (2005) point out that 'strategies to prevent and manage violence and aggression in the health care setting have become a primary health and safety issue.' They describe a program for preventing behavioural violence and aggression including staff education and training, risk assessment and management practices, and the use of patient contracts and policy development. Awalt *et al.* (1997) point out that 'levels of anger and violence are higher in substance abusers than in the general population.' Cork & Ferns (2008) highlight the prevalence of alcohol related violence, stating that 'violence in the emergency department (ED) is a global problem.'

The National Institute for Health and Clinical Excellence's (NICE, 2005) guidelines *The Short-Term Management of Disturbed/Violent Behaviour in In-Patient Psychiatric Setting and Emergency Department*

states that staff: 'should receive ongoing competency training to recognise anger, potential aggression, antecedents and risk factors of disturbed/violent behaviour, and to monitor their own verbal and non-verbal behaviour. Training should include methods of anticipating, deescalating or coping with disturbed/violent behaviour.'

Prediction of violence is difficult. The Guidelines states that clinician's judgement is only slightly better than chance. 'Antecedents/warning signs for the occurrence of disturbed/violent incidents include: verbal abuse, aggressive/agitated behaviour, threatening gestures and abnormal activity levels and staff limit-setting.' Steinert *et al.* (1991) state that 'conflicts between patients and staff precede aggressive incidents in the majority of cases.'

It is therefore important that staff are proficient in de-escalation techniques. Richter (2006) states that 'staff are undertrained and underequipped concerning nonphysical interventions.' Rew & Ferns (2005) state that the 'NHS Zero Tolerance Zone Campaign suggests that there are alternative and more effective, techniques in dealing with violence and aggression that can be used to defuse a situation before it ever becomes a physical altercation.' However, according to the NICE Guidelines (2005), 'the lack of evaluations of the effectiveness of training in a clinical environment mean that a "gold standard" training package for the short-term management of disturbed/violent behaviour in psychiatric in-patient settings cannot be determined.'

According to the NICE Guidelines (2005):

- De-escalation involves the use of techniques that calm down an escalating situation or service user; therefore, action plans should stress that de-escalation should be employed early on in any escalating situation.
- A service user's anger needs to be treated with an appropriate, measured and reasonable response.
- Staff should accept that in a crisis situation they are responsible for avoiding provocation. It is not realistic to expect the person exhibiting disturbed/violent behaviour to simply calm down.

- Staff should learn to recognise what generally and specifically upsets and calms people. This will involve listening to individual service users and carer's reports of what upsets the service user, and this should be reflected in the service user's care plan.
- Staff should be aware of, and learn to monitor and control, their own verbal and nonverbal behaviour, such as body posture and eye contact.
- Where possible and appropriate, service users should be encouraged to recognise their own trigger factors, early warning signs of disturbed/violent behaviour, and other vulnerabilities. This information should be included in care plans and a copy given to the service user. Service users should also be encouraged to discuss and negotiate their wishes should they become agitated.
- Where de-escalation techniques fail to sufficiently calm a situation or service user, staff should remember that verbal de-escalation is an ongoing element of the management of an escalating individual. Verbal de-escalation is supported but not replaced by appropriate physical intervention.

The NICE Guidelines (2005) gives more detail of de-escalation techniques:

One staff member should assume control of a potentially disturbed/ violent situation. The staff member who has taken control should:

- Consider which de-escalation techniques are appropriate for the situation;
- Manage others in the environment, for example removing other service users from the area, enlisting the help of colleagues and creating space;
- Explain to the service user and others in the immediate vicinity what they intend to do;
- Give clear, brief, assertive instructions;
- Move towards a safe place and avoid being trapped in a corner.

The staff member who has taken control should ask for facts about the problem and encourage reasoning. This will involve:

- Attempting to establish a rapport and emphasising cooperation;
- Offering and negotiating realistic options and avoiding threats;
- Asking open questions and inquiring about the reason for the service user's anger, for example 'What has caused you to feel upset/angry?'
- Showing concern and attentiveness through non-verbal and verbal responses;
- Listening carefully and showing empathy, acknowledging any grievances, concerns or frustrations, and not being patronising or minimising service user concerns.

The staff member who has taken control should ensure that their own nonverbal communication is nonthreatening and not provocative. This will involve:

- Paying attention to non-verbal cues, such as eye contact and allowing greater body space than normal adopting a non-threatening but safe posture;
- Appearing calm, self-controlled and confident without being dismissive or over-bearing.
- Where there are potential weapons, the disturbed/violent person should be relocated to a safer environment, where at all possible. Where weapons are involved, a staff member should ask for the weapon to be placed in a neutral location rather than handed over.
- Staff should consider asking the service user to make use of the designated area or room specifically for the purpose of reducing arousal and/or agitation to help them calm down. In services where seclusion is practised, the seclusion room should not routinely be used for this purpose.

Rew & Ferns (2005) point out that 'the philosophies of eastern martial arts can teach us a lot about personal self-esteem and confidence which are two key elements in managing conflict situations.'

Rocca *et al.* (2006) state that 'the assessment of a violent patient may be very difficult due to the lack of a full medical and psychiatric history and the non-cooperativeness of the patient.' Their view is that:

The primary task and the short term outcome in a behavioural emergency is to act as soon as possible to stop the violence from escalating and to find the quickest way to keep the patient's agitation and violence under control with the maximum of safety for everybody and using the less severe effective intervention. Based on rather limited evidence, a wide variety of medications for the pharmacological treatment of acute aggression has been recommended: typical and atypical antipsychotics and benzodiazepines.

The NICE Guidelines (2005) states that 'the body of evidence suggests rapid tranquillisation as an intervention for the short-term management of disturbed/violent behaviour is both reasonably effective and reasonably safe. This evidence suggests that both benzodiazepines and antipsychotics appear to be effective and reasonably safe for use in rapid tranquillisation.'

Although physical restraint and seclusion are used relatively frequently in the in-patient psychiatric setting, the NICE Guidelines (2005) states that 'there is insufficient evidence to determine the effectiveness and safety of either physical interventions or seclusion for the short-term management of disturbed/violent behaviour in psychiatric in-patient settings.'

Bonner & McLaughlin (2007) draw attention to the fact that 'the psychological impact of aggression remains an area of concern. Post-incident review has been identified as an approach to considering untoward incidents of aggression, yet post-incident support and interventions for staff experiencing the psychological effects of aggression remain inconsistent and curtailed in many areas.'

Patients with mental health problems

Hargie & Dickson (2004) point out that 'it is difficult to listen to a very slow speaker. Professionals who have to deal with depressed clients will be aware of the problems involved in maintaining concentration with someone who says very little. At the other extreme, it is difficult to listen effectively for an extended period to a very rapid speaker, since we cannot handle the volume of information being received.' Sometimes it is helpful to comment on the speed of speech, to ask the patient if they have noticed that they are slower than usual, or whether they are finding that the thoughts are coming so quickly that their speech can barely keep up with them.

A patient may be finding it very difficult to say anything at all. Maguire (2000) states that 'most withdrawn patients will acknowledge that they are indeed finding it difficult to get into conversation. You should then ask why they are finding it difficult.' He suggests a number of ways of drawing the patient out:

- 'I get the feeling that we are finding it difficult to get into a discussion about your problems.'
- 'I have to work with the part of you that is willing to try and confront your problems so that I can see if we can do anything about them.'

Even if a person is depressed, psychotic, or intent on self-destruction, there is often a part, albeit small, that wants to keep safe and get better. If you can enlist the help of this part then you can start a dialogue.

When you attempt to take a history, a person will sometimes say: 'I'm not going through all that again. I'm fed up of talking, it doesn't do any good anyway.'

Then you might say: 'Ok, that's fine, I've understood some of what has been happening. You don't need to say anything. Let me talk to you for a few minutes, then we can see what you think.' This allows the person to dictate the pace, while still articulating the fact that you do expect something to be said at some point. By the time they have listened to you for five or ten minutes, they will probably be happy to talk. You can use this time to empathise with his predicament, to express how sorry you are that things have been difficult, and that you have some ideas about things that might be helpful and would like, with their permission, to talk about those too.

Tomm (1998) states that 'even withdrawn and / or mute clients find it difficult to escape entering into a process of silent conversing when questions are addressed to them.'

They may find that something the doctor says resonates with what they were feeling, and sometimes a person asking questions can put things in a new perspective or help people to understand contributing factors. Furthermore, they may realise that others do understand something of what they are going through.

It is not only people with a known mental health problem who may be suffering from psychological disorder. There are many people who are physically ill who have unrecognised symptoms. Maguire (2000) states that 'about 25–30% of patients with chronic disabling or serious life-threatening illness will develop clinical anxiety or depression. These disorders can result in the patient becoming very irritable, despairing and difficult to reassure.' In addition, patients with unexplained physical symptoms have high rates of psychological symptoms. For instance, Van Hemert (1993) found that the prevalence of psychiatric disorders was 15% for patients with a medical explanation for their presenting symptom, and 38–45% for patients with ill-explained or unexplained symptoms.

The RCP report (1997) states that:

> *Some illnesses are difficult to diagnose, explain or manage. A patient may have a predominantly physical basis for his or her complaint, but commonly the psycho-social component dominates. In either case, their illness exerts a profound psychological effect, and management that does not take account of a patient's understanding and fears is bound to be incomplete. Doctors sometimes fail to pick up the clues to underlying psychological problems which contribute in part or in whole to the patient's illness.*

Complaints

The Royal College of Physicians (1997) report that 'complaints by patients about the treatment they receive are increasing in frequency and most of these can be laid at the door of failures of communication. Whatever the cause, once a complaint has occurred, dealing with it satisfactorily requires good communication skills.'

Dyer (2009) states that 'the 2008 fitness to practise statistics show that the number of doctors complained about to the General Medical Council rose by 32% between 2002 and 2008, from 4452 doctors in

2002 to 5195 in 2008. Greater numbers of complaints occur against doctors who qualified outside the United Kingdom or Europe.'

Groene *et al.* (2009) conducted a survey of 351 European hospital managers and professionals, and found that:

> *hospitals reported high implementation of policies for patients' rights (85.5%) and informed consent (93%), whereas strategies to involve patients (71%) and learn from their experience (66%) were less frequently implemented. For 13 out of 18 hospital strategies, institutions with a more developed quality improvement system consistently reported better results.'*

However, such systems seemed to be 'insufficient to ensure widespread implementation of patient-centredness throughout the organisation (Groene *et al.*, 2009).'

Szewczyk (2007) point out that 'to reveal medical errors is regarded as the most efficient method of decreasing their number and of creation of the culture of patients' safety.' Yet Gallagher *et al.* (2006) report studies that suggest that 'less than half of harmful errors are disclosed to patients.' From reviewing the literature, they found that 'following errors, patients want an explicit statement that an error has occurred, information about why the error happened, how recurrences will be prevented, and an apology.' However, the study by Gallagher *et al.* (2006) which used clinical scenarios to investigate how physicians disclose errors to patients in the United States and Canada showed that:

> *56% chose statements that mentioned the adverse event but not the error, while 42% would explicitly state that an error occurred. Some physicians disclosed little information: 19% would not volunteer any information about the error's cause, and 63% would not provide specific information about preventing future errors. While all the scenarios involved clear-cut serious errors, many physicians would not explicitly apologize.*

The Royal College of Physicians (1997) state that 'feelings of regretful sympathy for suffering can and should be expressed even where a complaint may be unjustified or where no one is at fault. A doctor who says that he or she is sorry that a patient has suffered is not admitting liability and should not fear possible litigation in simply expressing sympathy or regret.' MacDonald (2004) reports that 'when mistakes have been made patients need to know the exact nature and scale of the error. They need to know the possible implications and long-term effects of such a mistake. They need to know how it came about that the mistake was made and what steps have been put in place to prevent the same error occurring again.'

Groopman (2008) makes the point that 'as many as 15% of all diagnoses are inaccurate, according to a 1995 report in which all doctors assessed written descriptions of patients' symptoms and examined actors simulating patients with various diseases. These findings match classical research, which shows that 10% to 15% of all diagnoses are wrong.' In which case, it seems a good idea to take a humble approach towards errors. 'Much will depend on adopting a constructive attitude to criticism rather than regarding it as a personal attack against which a defence has to be mounted' (RCP, 1997). As MacDonald (2004) states, 'patients usually understand that mistakes are difficult to report, and respect the doctor who can manage to explain promptly, sincerely and with a genuine acceptance of the need to learn from the mistake.'

Chapter 11
New directions

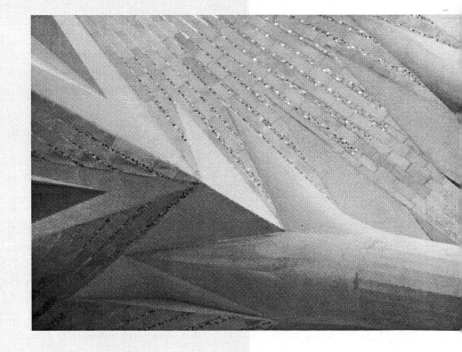

New directions

Looking after ourselves

The BMA News (Nov 14 2009) reported that the World Medical Association (WMA) urged the medical profession 'to remove the stigma surrounding burnout and called on governments to address the issue,' and states that 'doctors should not have to choose between saving themselves and serving their patients.' There is evidence that stigma continues to be a disincentive for doctors to acknowledge problems. For instance, Cohen *et al.* (2005) report that 'there are many anecdotal accounts of undergraduates and qualified doctors feeling that their progress will be tarnished if they acknowledge problems connected to stress, distress and communication.'

De Mercato *et al.* (1995) assessed the prevalence of the burnout syndrome in physicians, nurses, and ancillary medical workers, and found that, overall, 45.5% reported symptoms of burnout.

McManus *et al.* (2002) conducted a three-year longitudinal study of 331 UK doctors in which they assessed stress and the three components of burnout (emotional exhaustion, depersonalization, and low personal accomplishment). They found that 'emotional exhaustion and stress showed reciprocal causation: high levels of emotional exhaustion caused stress, and high levels of stress caused emotional exhaustion. High levels of personal accomplishment increased stress levels, whereas depersonalization lowered stress levels.'

Bub (2006) states that 'the life of a typical physician includes a spectrum of trauma that varies from chronic stress punctuated by moments of fear to acute catastrophic fright.' One of the ways that doctors may attempt to decrease the emotional impact and effort is to detach from their emotions when dealing with patients. As Ramirez *et al.* (1996) explain, depersonalisation means treating people in an unfeeling, impersonal way. Another way of dealing with stress is to deny its effects. Maguire (2000) makes the point that 'doctors appear to be more at risk of burnout if they believe that denial of their own personal needs is desirable or that their own uncertainties and emotions must be kept private.'

Pendleton *et al.* (2003) state that: 'doctors are as affected by emotional factors in their work as is any other professional.' Longhurst (1989) explains that:

> *it is a profound experience to confront, as a physician, the fears and trepidations of someone else's illness, which might include their pain, dying, birth, disfigurement, and loneliness. These emotionally charged issues can be addressed with greater sensitivity by the physician who has a sense of self. When physicians are better attuned, have that sense of self, they can make the connections essential to healing.*

Neighbour (2005) states that 'the self-awareness and self-care of doctors is important if they are to give the best therapeutic attention to patients. Part of professional competence is the ability to offer each successive patient a caring and compassionate state of mind uncontaminated with our personal preoccupations.' He puts forward the idea of 'housekeeping' – looking after your own internal experience. Turner (2001) makes the point that 'clinicians may be exhausted by the emotional needs of their patients ... they cannot provide excellent clinical care if they fail to nurture themselves physically, emotionally and spiritually.' It is important for each individual to find ways in which they can share burdens, obtain support, and process emotions.

Support and supervision

Supervision plays an important part in shaping doctors' attitudes and coping strategies. Senior doctors are powerful role models for trainees. Maguire (2000) makes the point that doctors 'also need to feel that they are cared for as individuals by their supervising colleagues, otherwise they will continue to use distancing strategies.' A trainee will learn to openly discuss emotions if their censultant encovrages. Recognition of problems and validation of feelings de-stigmatise. If a trainee can talk freely about them own emotional responses to patients, then it is likely that their they are able to respond to patients' feelings more effectively and sympathetically.

Novack *et al.* (1997) suggest 'organized activities that can promote physician personal awareness such as support groups, Balint groups, and discussions of meaningful experiences in medicine.

Experience with these activities suggests that through enhancing personal awareness physicians can improve their clinical care and increase satisfaction with work, relationships, and themselves.'

Maguire (2000) writes that 'the aim of Balint groups is to help doctors to identify blind spots in their attitudes and behaviour – that is, issues related to them becoming over- or under-involved with patients of which they were not previously aware.' Other types of reflective groups, if available, can be helpful, particularly if facilitated by a group analyst or psychotherapist.

Reflection

Each individual must find a place in which to reflect on the events, emotions, stresses and difficulties that have arisen in their own medical practice. In addition to verbal discussion with colleagues, it is useful to set aside some time for silent reflection. This can be either alone or with others. Meditation is increasingly recognised as a useful technique for creating this space and time.

A number of authors have researched the impact of meditation on stress. In the United States in 1979, Kabat-Zinn began teaching an eight-week Mindfulness Based Stress Reduction programme to help patients cope with stress, pain and illness. Mindfulness is calm awareness of one's physical sensations, feelings, content of consciousness, or consciousness itself.

Bishop (2002) explains that 'Mindfulness-Based Stress Reduction (MBSR) is a clinical program, developed to facilitate adaptation to medical illness, which provides systematic training in mindfulness meditation as a self-regulatory approach to stress reduction and emotion management. There has been widespread and growing use of this approach within medical settings in the last twenty years.' Salmon *et al.* (2004) state that: 'based in Buddhist philosophy and subsequently integrated into Western health care in the contexts of psychotherapy and stress management, mindfulness meditation is evolving as a systematic, clinical intervention.'

Various studies have shown the effects of meditation both in clinical populations and in healthy people. Schreiner & Malcolm (2008) suggest that 'mindfulness training is beneficial in reducing the symptoms of subclinical depression and anxiety and can substantially reduce stress.' Carmody & Baer (2008) found that 'eight sessions of MBSR increased levels of mindfulness and well-being and decreased stress and symptoms.' Chiesa & Serretti (2009) state that 'MBSR is able to reduce stress levels in healthy people. A meta-analysis of results from 55 studies indicated that some meditation practices produced significant changes in healthy participants (Ospina *et al.*, 2007). Mindfulness meditation techniques appear to reduce stress arousal (Epel *et al.*, 2009), and increases in mindfulness have been shown to mediate reductions in perceived stress and rumination (Shapiro *et al.*, 2008).

Greeson (2008) reviewed 52 studies into the effects of mindfulness on the mind, the brain, the body, and behaviour. He found that 'cultivating a more mindful way of being is associated with less emotional distress, more positive states of mind, and better quality of life. In addition, mindfulness practice can influence the brain, the autonomic nervous system, stress hormones, the immune system, and health behaviours.'

Praissman (2008) conducted a literature review which showed that 'both patients and healthcare providers experiencing stress or stress-related symptoms benefit from MBSR programs. They concluded that MBSR is a safe, effective, integrative approach for reducing stress, and that it is therapeutic for healthcare providers, enhancing their interactions with patients.'

There are, in addition, many other types of meditative practice. Different methods suit different people. For example, Pace *et al.* (2009) make the point that 'while much attention has been paid to meditation practices that emphasize calming the mind, improving focused attention, or developing mindfulness, less is known about meditation practices that foster compassion.' Their study found that 'engagement in compassion meditation may reduce stress-induced immune and behavioral responses.'

Meditation can decrease stress, help us to relax and find that inner peace which is within each of us. It is one way of achieving an expansion of consciousness, a greater awareness – of self and others. It can also awaken our inner observer, and allow us to know our own innermost thoughts and feelings.

Chapter 11

We, as doctors, are privileged to accompany patients along their path – through pain and suffering, through life and death. Intuitively, it makes sense that by looking after ourselves, we are better able to look after others. By opening our hearts and minds, we are better able to care.

Chapter 12

Learning points

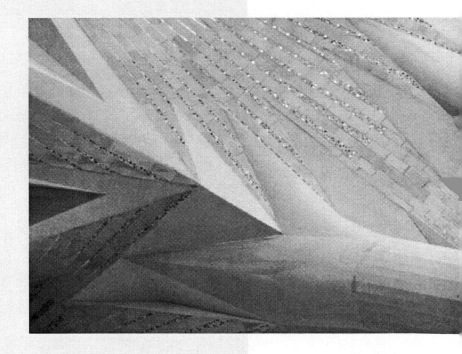

Learning points

Chapter 1: Introduction

Why do doctors need to communicate better?

As far back as 1968, Korsch (1968) found that 24% of patients reported dissatisfaction, notably due to lack of warmth and friendliness on the part of the doctor, failure to take into account the patient's concerns and expectations, lack of clear-cut explanation, and use of medical jargon.

> Communication difficulties are one of the main reasons that patients complain about doctors. The most common criticism is not about the doctor's competence but rather that he or she has failed either to listen or to offer sufficient explanation (RCP, 1997).

According to the BMA (2004), patients are less likely to complain or to sue if doctors communicate well.

> Problematic communication with patients is thought to contribute to emotional burnout and low personal accomplishment in doctors as well as high psychological morbidity (Feinman, 2002).

How the role of doctors is changing

The biomedical model, in which doctors have traditionally been trained, does not take adequate account of psychological and social factors which are not only relevant to chronic illness, but also are of increasing importance in the management of those rising numbers of patients for whom there is no medical diagnosis or physical explanation of symptoms.

> Healthcare is increasingly a partnership. The emphasis has shifted from a doctor-centred or disease-centred model to a patient-centred model, in which the patient is now much more involved in decisions.

Doctors are now expected to participate in management and leadership at all levels of their training and career, and this requires a different style of communication.

The changing NHS

The government White Paper *The NHS Plan 2000* heralded the beginning of a ten-year redirection of the NHS. This meant, as outlined in the core principles of the Plan, that patients would be treated as individuals; that partnerships would develop between patients and staff; and that patients would have more say in their own treatment.

The introduction of the European Working Time Directive has made a substantial impact on doctors' training and working lives.

Changes in demographics

In most developed countries, people are living longer, and as a result, disease patterns are changing. There are more chronic or long-term illnesses such as heart disease, stroke, cancer, arthritis, diabetes, mental illness, asthma and other conditions (*Expert Patient*, DH, 2001b).

Mental health problems have become much more prevalent: they are now the most frequent causes of sick leave, (Confederation of British Industry, 2005); they account for at least one in four GP consultations (NHS Plan, 2000), and it is estimated that they affect up to 20% of the child and adolescent population (*Expert Patient*, DH 2001b).

Medically unexplained symptoms, which are physical symptoms which have no medical diagnosis or explanation, are also increasing in prevalence. Nimnuan *et al.* (2000) looked at seven specialist clinics in one hospital and found that 51% of new patients were diagnosed as having medically unexplained symptoms (Reid *et al.*, 2001).

The NHS Constitution, published by the Department of Health in January 2009, sets out the principles and values of the NHS, including a commitment to high-quality care that is safe, effective and focused on patient experience. The Constitution reflects a changing ethos within healthcare provision. It states quite clearly that patients must participate in all decisions about treatment. In other words, the doctor is no longer expected to weigh the balance alone.

Traditional communication skills training

- A well known study of medical education found that medical students' interpersonal skills with patients declined as their medical education progressed (Helfer, 1970 in Roter & Hall, 2006).
- Paternalism is widely regarded as the traditional form of the doctor-patient relationship and it is still seen as the most common one (Emanuel & Emanuel, 1992; Roter & Hall, 2006).
- Without specific training in communication skills, medical students' ability to communicate deteriorates as they progress through their traditional medical training. They enter medical school with better communication skills than when they leave (Kurtz *et al.*, 2005).
- Traditionally, a medical approach to history-taking, based on the belief that every illness is caused by a disease with an external definable cause, has predominated. Taking a history in this formal and structured way tends to make consultations disease or doctor-centred (Thistlethwaite & Jordan, 1999).

The patient-centred approach

Stewart (2001) states that patients want patient-centred care which:

- explores the patients' main reason for the visit, concerns, and need for information; (b) seeks an integrated understanding of the patients' world–that is, their whole person, emotional needs, and life issues;
- finds common ground on what the problem is and mutually agrees on management;
- enhances prevention and health promotion;

- enhances the continuing relationship between the patient and the doctor.

Holman & Lorig (2000) make the point that when acute disease was the primary cause of illness, patients were generally inexperienced and passive recipients of medical care. Now that chronic disease has become the principal medical problem, the patient must become a co-partner in the process.

The new role of doctors

In 1981 only 30% of medical schools in the UK gave any teaching in communication skills (RCP, 1997). However, in 1993, the GMC emphasised the importance of the development of skills to interact with patients and colleagues (*Tomorrow's Doctors*, 1993), and many medical schools began to revise their teaching and assessment of communication skills (BMA, 2004).

Ten years later, *Tomorrow's Doctors* (2003) reinforced that graduates must be able to communicate clearly, sensitively and effectively with patients, relatives, and colleagues. *Tomorrow's Doctors* (2009) has now been published, and medical schools are preparing for its application from 2011/12 onwards.

In 2006, the GMC revised *Good Medical Practice* (first published 1995), which set the standards for doctors at both undergraduate and postgraduate levels. It stated the need for a good working relationship with patients, based on trust, openness and good communication (GMC, 2006).

Communication skills are now regarded as a core competence. Assessment of communication skills will be necessary as part of the doctor's appraisal and personal development plans (BMA, 2004).

The Medical Leadership Competency Framework (2008) states that all doctors and medical students must be actively involved in the planning, delivery and transformation of health services. Introduction of this Framework will have a significant impact on how doctors are trained. To be deemed an effective and safe doctor in the future, competence in both clinical and wider non-clinical competences including management and leadership will be required (Clark & Armit, 2008).

A *new philosophy*

Doctors are now observed, appraised, and rated on both clinical and, latterly, non-clinical skills. They have been expected to take on a gradually expanding range of non-clinical roles and responsibilities that their training has not prepared them for.

In 1994 it was found that the estimated prevalence of psychiatric morbidity was 27% among consultants in five specialties: gastroenterology, radiology, surgical oncology, clinical oncology, and medical oncology (Ramirez *et al.*, 1996). By 2002, in the same five specialties, it had risen to 32%, and the prevalence of emotional exhaustion had increased from 32% in 1994 to 41% in 2002.

Doctors have a very high incidence of alcoholism, depressive illness and chronic stress disorders (Tate, 2007), and, in the UK, the suicide rate for doctors is approximately twice the national average (Ramirez *et al.*, 1996).

Chapter 2: How doctors communicate

Research evidence on doctors' communication skills

In the UK in 1976, Byrne & Long analysed 2,500 patient visits, and published a paper which looked in depth for the first time at the way in which consultations in general practice were being conducted. They found that:

- Many doctors are not good listeners.
- The way in which a doctor sets about a consultation is largely repetitive.
- At least 20% of consultations show insensitivity on the part of the doctor.
- Many doctors feel hopeless when faced with a 'sick' patient who has nothing organic wrong.

- Few demonstrate the capacity to meet the needs of those patients whose problems do not fit into an organic disease pattern.

Beckman & Frankel in 1984 found that:

- Doctors allowed patients to complete their opening statement in only 23% of visits.
- In 51 (69%) of the visits, the physician interrupted the patient's opening statement – after a mean time of only 18 seconds – and directed questions toward a specific concern.
- Once patients had been interrupted, they were unlikely to disclose further concerns.
- In only one of these 51 visits was the patient able to return to, and complete, his or her opening statement, ie the concerns for which they sought care.
- Given sufficient time and opportunity, the patient will mark the end of his or her opening statement of concerns.
- When allowed to finish, no patient's opening statement took more than 150 seconds.

Beckman *et al.* (1985) found that doctors were taking control of the content of the interview too early in the visit, and were choosing one problem to explore rather than eliciting the patient's full agenda, In addition, they found that patients who completed their statement of concerns in the opening moments of the encounter were significantly less likely to raise concerns toward the end of the visit.

In 1999, Marvel *et al.* repeated the original study to find out whether behaviour had changed. They found that:

- Only 28% of experienced physicians solicited the patient's complete agenda.
- The mean time available to patients to initially express their concerns before the first physician redirection was 23.1 seconds.
- Most redirections (76%) occurred after the first concern.

- Once the discussion became focused on a specific concern, the likelihood of returning to complete the agenda was very low. Patient concerns were eventually completed in only 8% of the visits.
- Patients who initiated one or more concerns and were given the opportunity to complete their concerns used an average of only 32 seconds.
- Physicians trained in family therapy and communication skills more frequently solicited concerns fully, often by an open-ended question followed by nondirective facilitating utterances (eg 'Uh-huh' or 'What else?') Having heard the patient's agenda, the multiple concerns were then explicitly prioritised with the patient.
- Using a simple opening solicitation, such as 'What concerns do you have?' then asking 'Anything else?' repeatedly until a complete agenda has been identified appears to take 6 seconds longer than interviews in which the patient's agenda is interrupted.

What do patients want to talk to doctors about?

Levenstein *et al.* (1989) defined the patient's agenda in terms of ideas, expectations and feelings, and the doctor's agenda in terms of the correct diagnosis of the patient's complaints.

Patients often have more than one concern.

Stewart *et al.* in 1979 showed that 54% of patients' complaints and 45% of their concerns were not elicited.

Maguire *et al.* (1996a) found that only a minority of health professionals identified more than 60% of their patients' main concerns.

White *et al.* (1994) found that 21% of patients in primary care introduced new problems, not previously discussed, in the closing moments of the medical visit.

> Beckman & Frankel (1989) quote various studies which have shown that 'patients are more satisfied during the interview when they have an opportunity to share their opinions (Stewart *et al.*, 1984), to ask questions (Roter, 1977), and when doctors show warmth (Francis *et al.*, 1969) and empathy (Wasserman *et al.*, 1984).'

Starfield *et al.* (1981) found that agreement leads to better outcomes and problem resolution, yet in 50% of visits the patient and the doctor did not agree on the nature of the presenting problem.

What do doctors want patients to talk about?

> The doctor's agenda is directed towards finding out enough relevant medical information from the patient in order to make the right diagnosis.

Peterson *et al.* (1992) found that in 61 out of 80 medical outpatients (76%), the history led to the final diagnosis.

> Langewitz *et al.* (1998) found that only 55 to 69% of medical information was identified by internal medicine residents during medical consultations.

Roter & Hall (2006) found that during medical visits the average amount of physician contribution to the medical dialogue is 60%, whereas patients contribute 40%.

> Stewart (1985) concluded that doctors who had mastered the patient-centred approach took little extra time compared with doctors who did not employ these techniques.

How much do patients want to be involved in decision-making?

Levinson *et al.* (2005) undertook a population-based study which showed that people vary substantially in how involved they wish to be in decisions about their care. They found that those over

45 years of age, and those in poorer health, tended to prefer a physician-directed style of decision-making.

McKinstry (2000) points out, however, that doctors need to determine for individual patients how much involvement in decision-making they want.

Waitzkin (1985) revealed that doctors spent little time informing their patients, overestimated the time they did spend and underestimated patients' desire for information.

Kindelan & Kent (1987) found that patients most wanted information about the diagnosis, prognosis and causation of their condition. Doctors greatly overestimated their desire for information about treatment and drug therapy (Silverman *et al.* , 2005).

What is good communication?

Growing evidence suggests that doctors who focus on the patient as well as the disease obtain more accurate historical data, increase patient adherence, and build more effective patient-physician relationships (Platt *et al.*, 2001).

Good communication helps the patient to recall information and comply with treatment instructions, and leads to improved patient satisfaction (Hulsman, 2002; Maguire & Pitceathly, 2002).

Better communication and dialogue has a beneficial effect in promoting better emotional health, resolution of symptoms and pain control (Meryn, 1998).

Change is more likely if patients are helped to make decisions for themselves rather than being told what to do (Rollnick *et al.*, 2005).

The Bristol Inquiry urged doctors to include patients as active participants in their own care, and to:

- Involve patients (or their parents) in decisions
- Keep patients (or parents) informed
- Provide patients with counselling and support
- Gain informed consent for all procedures and processes
- Elicit feedback from patients and listen to their views
- Be open and candid when adverse events occur (Coulter, 2002a).

DiMatteo & Chow (1995) suggest the following steps for enhancing compliance and improving communication:

1. Explain to patients their diagnosis and possible causes.
2. Listen to the patient's fears and frustrations. Encourage patients to ask questions and to describe personal expectations for treatment, including effects on lifestyle.
3. Answer patient's questions. Address unrealistic expectations.
4. Suggest a treatment approach that may fit the patient's expressed preferences. Describe expected benefits and costs, risks, and expected outcomes, and other possible courses of action, including no treatment.
5. Obtain patient feedback concerning benefits of treatment along with understanding and acceptance of risk. Devise methods to address concerns.
6. Discuss with the patient in detail when and how medication will be taken. Correct misunderstandings.
7. Work with the patient to elicit commitment to following the treatment regimen. If the patient appears hesitant, return to step 2. Simplifying and reminding will not help a patient follow a regimen that he or she does not believe in.
8. Work with the patient to build supports for and reduce barriers to the regimen.
9. Revisit the issue of when and how the regimen will implemented, and attempt to anticipate problems and suggest solutions.

What is poor communication?

Ley (1988) points out that patients often do not understand or remember what they are told. What clinicians say is often not in understandable or memorable form.

There is evidence that many physicians listen poorly, miss vital non-verbal cues, misdiagnose emotional and mental conditions, and respond with a lack of understanding and insight (Bub, 2006).

Heath (1984) showed that when doctors attempt to read the patient's records and listen to the patient at the same time, they frequently miss or forget what the patient tells them.

The Royal College of Physicians (1997) reports a variety of reasons for poor communication, including: the inability of doctors to recognise patients' concerns; the tendency to overlook the need of patients to be heard and to be given clear explanations, and the failure to take psychological and social factors into account.

Patient satisfaction

Korsch (1989) defines satisfaction, for both patient and doctor, as a short-term outcome of the medical interaction which can be measured immediately following an encounter.

A Consumers' Association survey of people who had made a first visit to see a hospital consultant revealed that about 85% were satisfied with what they had been told by the specialist, and of those about 50% were very satisfied (RCP, 1997).

Patient satisfaction is also related to the amount of information that patients are given.

Meryn (1998): Patients want more and better information about their problem and the outcome, more openness about the side effects of treatment, relief of pain and emotional distress, and advice on what they can do for themselves.

Providing information has also been shown to be associated with improved resolution of symptoms, reduced emotional distress, improved physiological status, reduced use of analgesia, reduced length of hospital stay, and improved quality of life (Kaplan *et*

al., 1989; Fallowfield *et al.*, 1994; Roter *et al.*, 1995; Stewart, 1995; Kinnersley *et al.*, 2008).

Hall *et al.* (1988) in a meta-analysis reported that patient satisfaction was related most dramatically to the amount of information given by doctors. It was also related to greater technical and interpersonal competence, more partnership building, more immediate and positive nonverbal behaviour, more social conversation, more positive talk, less negative talk and more communication overall.

Jackson *et al.* (2001) quote studies which have shown that patients rate health outcomes of care as the most important determinant of satisfaction.

However, various researchers express reservations about the reliability of satisfaction data because it is known that patients are reluctant to be critical (Jackson *et al.*, 2001, Shilling *et al.*, 2003) and are sometimes fearful of provoking a worsening of their care (Shilling *et al.*, 2003).

Patient compliance/concordance

The term concordance, introduced in 1997 by the Royal Pharmaceutical Society, was incorporated into the *Expert Patient* (DH, 2001b) and endorsed by the Department of Health in 2002. The principles were that doctors should provide clear and sufficiently detailed information to patients in order that the wishes of the patient can be incorporated into the process of prescribing (Heath, 2003).

According to the *Expert Patient* (DH, 2001b), concordance is an agreement reached after negotiation between a patient and a healthcare professional. Doctor and patient discuss why treatment is needed and what options are available. The doctor explores the patient's preferences, and finds out what the patient has learned about the consequences of taking or not taking prescribed medications.

Elwyn *et al.* (2003) state that doctors often do not name the drug they prescribe, or describe how new drugs differ from those previously prescribed; they do not usually check patients' understanding, explore their concerns, or discuss patients' ability to follow a treatment plan.

Coulter (2002b) reports that there is little evidence that general practitioners and patients share decision-making.

If the patient is not fully convinced that the medication is necessary and that the benefits will outweigh the risks, then it is quite likely that they will not take it as directed.

It is important to ask questions such as; 'Have you been taking the medication? Are there times when you forget it? What influences whether you take it or not? Is there anything else you need to know in order to decide whether this medication is the best treatment for you?'

Around one-third of people in the United Kingdom receive long-term medication (Dowell *et al.*, 2002). However, it is well known that many patients do not take the medicines prescribed. The figure of 50% suggested by Haynes *et al.* (1996) is often quoted as a typical rate of adherence.

The Royal College of Physicians (1997) states that inadequate explanation is the most frequent cause of poor compliance, as patients may be unwilling or unable to comply with suggested treatments if they do not understand the reasons for what has been proposed.

Providers who have a controlling, paternalistic manner give patients little opportunity to make a personal commitment to the regimen (DiMatteo *et al.*, 1995).

As the NICE guidance (2009) states, the patient has the right to decide not to take a medicine, even if the doctor does not agree with the decision, as long as the patient has the capacity to make an informed decision and has been provided with the necessary information.

Patients at greatest risk for non-adherence to treatment include: those who are most severely ill with serious diseases (DiMatteo *et al.*, 2007); those from families in conflict (DiMatteo, 2004b); and those who are depressed (DiMatteo *et al.*, 2000).

Dowell *et al.* (2002) identified four problematic issues for patients using treatment suboptimally: understanding, acceptance, level of personal control, and motivation. Identifying and discussing these barriers improved management for some.

Health outcomes

Levinson *et al.* (2005) quote various studies which show that 'patients who are knowledgeable about their condition (Kaplan *et al.*, 1989; Greenfield *et al.* 1985: Greenfield *et al.* 1988), or are involved in decision-making (Deber *et al.*, 996) enjoy improved health outcomes.'

Effective communication skills have been correlated to positive outcomes such as adherence to therapy, understanding of treatment risks (Travaline *et al.*, 2005); biological outcomes in chronic disease, and patient satisfaction (Levinson & Lurie, 2004).

Patients who ask questions, elicit treatment options, express opinions, and state preferences about treatment have measurably better health outcomes than patients who do not (Kaplan *et al.*, 1989).

Patients who feel that they have participated in decision-making are more likely to follow through on those decisions than those who do not (Kaplan *et al.*, 1996).

Stewart (1995) reviewed randomised controlled trials and found that:

In 16 of 21 studies the quality of communication both in the history-taking and discussion of the management plan influenced patient health outcomes. The outcomes affected were, in descending order of frequency, emotional health, symptom resolution, function, physiologic measures (ie blood pressure and blood sugar level) and pain control.

Coulter *et al.* (1999) quote various studies investigating the benefits of shared decision-making:

- Patients with hypertension benefit if they are allowed to adopt an active rather than a passive role in treatment (England & Evans, 1992).
- Patients with breast cancer suffer less depression and anxiety if they are treated by doctors who adopt a participative consultation style (Fallowfield *et al.*, 1990).
- Patients who are more actively involved in discussion about the management of their diabetes achieve better blood sugar control (Kaplan *et al.*, 1989).

Shilling *et al.* (2003) report various studies on cancer diagnosis which showed that women who were not satisfied with the information given at time of diagnosis adjusted less well to their cancer and its treatment (Fallowfield, 1990), and that patients who rated their doctors' discussion of treatment options highly had better psychological adjustment to a cancer diagnosis (Butow *et al.*, 1996).

In a review of evidence on patient- doctor communication, Stewart *et al.* (1999) found that the following aspects of communication about the management plan significantly influenced health outcomes:

- Patient being encouraged to ask questions.
- Provision of clear information.
- Willingness of doctor to share decision-making.
- Agreement between patient and doctor about the problem and the plan.

Medical failure

Richards (1990) states that 'most complaints by patients and the public about doctors deal with problems of communication not with clinical competency.'

Coulter (2002a) states that, in addition, 'failure to take account of the patient's perspective is at the heart of most formal complaints and legal actions.'

Frenkel & Liebman (2004), former litigators and now mediators and clinical law teachers, state that 'ineffective communication is the single largest factor in producing patient litigation and good communication, including effective apologies, can avert or help end conflict, especially litigation. Apologies have a potential for healing that is matched only by the difficulty most people have in offering them.'

Irwin & Richardson (2006) quote Beckman *et al.* (2004) who conducted a study of malpractice cases against a metropolitan medical centre. They found that problematic relationship issues between the doctor and patient were identified in 71% of the depositions. These could be categorized by four themes:

- deserting the patient (32%),
- devaluing patient and/or family views (29%),
- delivering information poorly (26%),
- failing to understand the patient and/or family perspective (13%).

If more attention had been focused on the physician/patient interaction, particularly at the post-outcome consultation, litigation could have been avoided in many of these cases.

Chapter 3: Communication theory

Language, says Groopman (2008), is still the bedrock of clinical practice. Communication is not simply a uni-directional flow, the delivery of a message or a set of instructions. It is a bilateral interaction in which physician and patient discuss the options and weigh the choices (Levinson *et al.*, 2005). It is a means of establishing and developing relationships – with patients and also with colleagues and other members of the healthcare team.

Littlejohn & Foss (2005) write that 'relationships consist of cybernetic patterns of interaction in which individuals' words and actions affect how others respond. We continually adapt our behaviours to the feedback from others, and in a relationship, both parties are doing this simultaneously.'

Berry (2007) makes the point that doctors and patients have very different views on the most important quality of a good doctor: Paling (2004) found that for doctors, it is diagnostic ability, whereas for patients it is listening. Doctors rated listening as least important.

Verbal and nonverbal communication

Tate (2007) pointed out that, looking at video recordings of consultations, it is surprising how often doctors do not seem to be very interested in their patient as an individual.

Heath (1984) found that patients use gestures to try to regain eye contact if the doctor has looked away.

Ruusuvuori (2001) found that patients find it problematic when doctors start reading or writing in the medical records, as they are not sure whether the doctor is still listening.

Platt *et al.* (2001) state that 'to be truly patient-centred, physicians must demonstrate both verbally and nonverbally that the most important part of the medical interview is the person facing them.'

Bull (2001) points out, 'nonverbal cues appear to be more important than speech in judgements of rapport. Nonverbal communication has sometimes been regarded as a kind of language of emotion and interpersonal relationships.'

Mehrabian (1972): 'if the verbal message is being contradicted by the nonverbal message, then the nonverbal message carries most weight.'

Griffiths *et al.* (2003) quote Nardone *et al.* (1992) who write that nonverbal cues 'may be less susceptible to censorship than verbal cues and therefore may be more reliable indicators of what is being communicated.'

Communication skills training

It is thought that in a forty-year career a doctor will conduct between 150,000 and 200,000 interviews with patients and their families.

Fallowfield *et al.* (2002) point out that very few doctors have received much formal training in communication, and the training provided is commonly inadequate.

Aspegren (1999) stated that 'the teaching method should be experiential as it has been shown conclusively that instructional methods do not give desired results. The content of communication skills courses should primarily be problem defining. Men are slower learners of communication skills than women, which should be taken into account by course organizers.'

Maguire & Pitceathly (2002) suggest that communication skills training should include three components of learning: cognitive input, modelling, and practice of key skills.

- Cognitive input: This includes education, discussion, and the examination and challenging of beliefs that may be restricting or limiting the possibilities for change. Seven types of communication problems were identified: 1) lack of trust/agreement, 2) too many problems, 3) feeling distressed, 4) lack of understanding, 5) lack of adherence, 6) demanding/controlling patient, and 7) special problems.
- Modelling: Langewitz *et al.* (1998) taught a behaviourally oriented intervention to residents in Internal Medicine

> for 22.5 hours over a 6-month period. They found that it was useful for participants to see themselves in video feedback; to try alternative behaviours once the problem had been identified; and to define individual goals after the workshop.
>
> - Practice of key skills: It appears that doctors find it difficult to transfer learned skills and behaviours into clinical practice (Langewitz *et al.*, 1998; Maguire & Pitceathly, 2002). Individual skills need to be practised until they can be comfortably and effectively used. Two examples are negotiating and taking up emotions.

Haskard *et al.* (2008) report that communication skills training for doctors improved patients' satisfaction with 'information and overall care; increased physicians' counselling (as reported by patients) about weight loss, exercise, and quitting smoking and alcohol; and increased independent ratings of physicians' sensitive, connected communication with their patients.'

Chapter 4: Communication skills

> This chapter looks at a number of ways of structuring the medical interview with a view to highlighting the specific communication skills required at each step.

Little *et al.* (2001a) stated that 'from the patient's perspective there are probably at least three important and distinct domains of patient-centredness: communication, partnership, and health promotion.'

> Campion *et al.* (2002) quote Mead & Bower (2000) who state that 'patient centeredness comprises five dimensions: a biopsychosocial perspective, the patient-as-person, sharing power and responsibility, the therapeutic alliance, and the doctor-as-person.'

The report of the Royal College of Physicians (1997) presents a model modified from Morris & Schofield (1992) which provides a checklist of steps needed for a successful and satisfying consultation:

- Relationship: establishes an effective relationship with the patient and demonstrates respect for the patient as a person.
- Structuring: conducts the consultation in a sequence logical to that particular patient's needs, and lets the patient know and follow the sequence, so that time is used effectively.
- History: elicits the patient's history and symptoms, their chronology and related factors, sufficiently to establish their possible causes.
- Question style: demonstrates the appropriate use of open, closed and reflective questions.
- Listening: listens to the patient and responds to cues.
- Patient's understanding and ideas: explores the patient's understanding and ideas about the nature and cause of the problems and their management.
- Patient's worries and concerns: explores and responds to the patient's worries and concerns about the problems and their management.
- Explaining: offers the patient an appropriate explanation of the problems and their management which is related to the patient's own ideas.
- Checking: checks that the patient understands any explanations and that concerns have been addressed.
- Involving: takes opportunities to involve the patient in the decision-making and his or her own management.

Langewitz *et al.* (1998) suggest specific interviewing skills:

- Help the patient clarify his/her concerns.
- Find relevant information.
- Offer a negotiation process.
- Invite patient participation in decision-making.
- Empathy in greeting behavior.
- Acknowledging initial complaints.
- Take up emotions instead of suppressing them.
- Clarify consultation reasons.
- Summarising patient's statement in doctor's own words.
- Summarising, acknowledging initial complaints, clarify purpose of the consultation.

- Explicit announcement of history-taking phase.
- Generally structuring the consultation.
- Shared evaluation of the consultation.
- Convey information as detailed as possible and as desired by the patient, ie results and preliminary diagnosis, aetiology, prognosis; communicate about treatment options, feasibility of treatment, future prospects.

Maguire & Pitceathly (2002) identify the following key tasks in communication with patients:

- Eliciting (a) the patient's main problems; (b) the patient's perceptions of these; and (c) the physical, emotional, and social impact of the patient's problems on the patient and family.
- Tailoring information to what the patient wants to know; checking his or her understanding.
- Eliciting the patient's reactions to the information given and his or her main concerns.
- Determining how much the patient wants to participate in decision-making (when treatment options are available).
- Discussing treatment options so that the patient understands the implications.
- Maximising the chance that the patient will follow agreed decisions about treatment and advice about changes in lifestyle.

Silverman *et al.* (2005) take the view that 'building the relationship and structuring the interview are tasks that occur throughout the interview rather than sequentially. Both of these continuous tasks are essential for the five sequential tasks to be completed successfully.'

Building the relationship includes:

- Appropriate nonverbal behaviour; eye contact, facial expression, posture, position, movement, vocal cues;
- If reads, writes notes or uses computer, does so in a manner that does not interfere with dialogue or rapport;
- Demonstrates appropriate confidence;

- Develops rapport; accepts, is not judgemental; uses empathy; overtly acknowledges patient's views and feelings;
- Provides support, offers partnership;
- Deals sensitively with embarrassing and disturbing topics and physical pain;
- Involving the patient: shares thinking, explains rationale and, during physical examination, explains process.

Providing structure to the consultation includes:

- Making organisation overt; summarises at the end of a specific line of enquiry;
- Progresses from one section to another using signposting and transitional statements; includes rationale for next section;
- Attending to flow: structures interview in logical sequence;
- Attends to timing and keeping interview on task.

Opening the session

Lipkin (1996) mentions that preparing the environment is an important first step in the consultation process; making sure that there is a quiet, comfortable, and private place in which you can interview the patient. The next step is preparing oneself by eliminating distractions, having a means of focusing the mind, through meditation or constructive imaging, and letting intrusive thoughts pass.

Kalet *et al.* (2004) also recommend that preparation includes review of the patient's notes, and an assessment of your own personal issues (values, biases and assumptions) going into the encounter.

The consultation is then opened by greeting the patient, introducing oneself, and inviting the patient to make himself comfortable. It may be useful at this point to explain your role, and to say how much time is available for the consultation. You can then go on to establish the reason for the patient's visit, outline an agenda, and make a personal connection (Makoul, 2001).

223

Gathering information and questioning

This section of the interview focuses on 'question/answer framing, working from open to closed questions, reflecting questions, silence without interruption, facilitation, response to verbal and non-verbal cues, clarification, summarising, and the negotiation of plans' (RCP, 1997).

Keller & Carroll (1994) state that patients have questions that they do not always ask, and that doctors should assume that they want to know:

1.   What has happened to me?
2.   Why has it happened to me?
3.   What is going to happen to me, in the short term, in the long-term?

They also advise doctors to answer questions about their actions, and to assume that patients want to know:

1.   What are you doing to me (examination, tests)?
2.   Why are you doing this rather than something else?
3.   Will it hurt me or harm me, for how long and how much?
4.   When and how will you know what these tests mean?
5.   When and how will I know what these tests mean?

Shilling *et al.* (2003) found that 'patient satisfaction was influenced by the simple act of asking if they have any questions during the consultation and by trying to ensure that the patient does not leave with unanswered questions.'

Platt *et al.* (2001) outline five areas of concern in getting to know the patient as a person:

•   Who is this patient? What constitutes that person's life? What are the patient's interests, work, important relationships, major concerns?
•   What does this patient want from the physician? What are their values and fears? What do they hope to accomplish here today or in the long run?

- How does this patient experience this illness? Specifically, what has it done to him functionally; how has it affected relationships; and what symbolic meaning does it hold for him?
- What are the patient's ideas about the illness? What is their understanding and perception of the disorder and its cause? What would seem to be reasonable treatment for it?
- What are the patient's main feelings about the illness, with special attention to the five common responses: fear, distrust, anger, sadness, and ambivalence?

Coulter *et al.* (1999) suggest that patients frequently would like the answers to these questions:

- Is it essential to have treatment for this problem?
- Will the treatment(s) relieve the symptoms?
- How long will it take to recover?
- What are the possible side effects?
- What effect will the treatment(s) have on my feelings and emotions?
- What effect will the treatment(s) have on my sex life?
- What do my carers need to know?
- What can I do to speed recovery?
- What are the options for rehabilitation?
- How can I prevent recurrence or future illness?
- Where can I get more information about the problem or treatments?

Explanation and planning

It is important to explain to the patient in easily understandable language what you are going to do, and the reasons for doing it, during a physical examination or procedure, or if further investigations are needed.

Silverman *et al.* (2005) state that the aims with explanation are to give comprehensive and appropriate information; to assess each individual patient's information needs; to neither restrict nor overload. To this end they suggest the doctor:

- Chunks and checks; gives information in assimilable chunks; checks for understanding; uses patients response as a guide to how to proceed;
- Assesses patient's starting point; asks for patient's prior knowledge; discovers extent of patient's wish for information;
- Asks patient what other information would be helpful;
- Gives explanation at appropriate times, not prematurely;
- Uses repetition and summarising: encourages patients to contribute;
- Negotiates a mutually acceptable plan; checks patient's concerns have been addressed.

Closing the session

At the end of the session, it is a good idea to briefly summarise the plan, and ask if the patient has any questions or other issues to discuss. Kalet states that, having arrived at a mutually acceptable solution, it is sensible to check the patient's willingness and ability to follow the plan. Then, clarify what to do in the interim, establish a safety net, schedule the next encounter and say goodbye (Lipkin, 1996).

Chapter 5: How to improve communication

Guidelines for good communication strategy (Royal College of Physicians, 1997):

- Provide the most important information first – good before bad.
- Explain how each item of information will affect the patient personally.
- Present information in separate categories.
- Make advice specific, detailed and concrete
- Use words the patients knows, or define unfamiliar words. Write down key words and unfamiliar words, draw a diagram, and keep a copy.
- Repeat the information, using the same words each time and prepare material, written or taped, to back up the handwritten note.

Pendleton *et al.* (2003) state that the MRCP includes a communication skills and ethics station in their clinical examination with the following criteria:

1. Communication skills – conduct of the interview
    *   introduces self to patient and explains role clearly
    *   agrees the purpose of the interview with the patient
    *   puts the patient at ease and establishes good rapport
    *   explores the patient's concerns, feelings and expectations – demonstrates empathy, respect, and non-judgemental attitude
    *   prioritises problems and redirects the interview sensitively
2. Communication skills – exploration and problem negotiation
    *   Appropriate questioning style – generally open-ended to closed a the interview progresses
    *   Provides clear explanations (jargon free) that the patient understands
    *   Agrees a clear course of action
    *   Summarises and checks the patient's understanding
    *   Concludes the interview appropriately
3. Ethics and law
    *   In relation to the clinical scenario, the candidates demonstrate knowledge of the relevant ethical and legal principles and appropriate attitudes in making decisions
    *   Knowledge of ethical principles
    *   Understanding of legal constraints applicable to the case
    *   Provides adequate reasoning as appropriate to the case.

The patient-centred approach: a model for clinical interviewing

The term 'patient-centred medicine' was introduced by Balint *et al.* in 1970 who contrasted it with 'illness-centred medicine.'

Byrne and Long (1976) reported that:

> *the patient-centred method is characterised by use of the patient's knowledge and experience; the doctor uses silence, listening and reflecting; clarifying and interpreting. This method stems from a belief in the ability of the patient to make decisions and to be involved in his own treatment.*
> *The doctor-centred method uses the doctor's skill and special knowledge; gathering information, analyzing and probing.*

Little *et al.* (2001a) found that 'patients in primary care strongly want a patient-centred approach, with communication, partnership, and health promotion.'

Patient-centred consulting has been shown to increase patient satisfaction (Kinnersley *et al.*, 1999), enhance outcomes of care including:

- Patient adherence to treatment recommendations
- Biological outcomes in chronic disease (Kaplan *et al.*, 1989; Levinson & Lurie, 2004)
- Increase the efficiency of care by reducing diagnostic tests and referrals (Stewart *et al.*, 2000).

Empathy

So what is empathy? According to Disiker & Michielutte (1981) it is 'the ability to understand what another person is experiencing and to communicate that understanding to the person.'

Stewart *et al.* (2000) state that 'psychosocial and psychiatric problems are common in general medical practice, but these diagnoses are missed in up to 50% of cases (Schulberg & Burns, 1988; Freeling *et al.*, 1985).'

Even as far back as 1957, Balint recognised that 'at least one-quarter to one-third of the work of the general practitioner consists of psychotherapy pure and simple.'

According to Coulehan *et al.* (2001):

> *numerous investigators have demonstrated the importance of empathy in the medical encounter. Empathy allows the patient to feel understood, respected and validated. This promotes diagnostic accuracy, therapeutic adherence, and patient satisfaction, while remaining time-efficient. Empathy also enhances physician satisfaction.*

Keller & Carroll (1994) note that empathy conveys an impression that the physician is 'present' and 'with' the patient.

In order to be present, the doctor must be focused on the patient, and emotionally available. Matthews *et al.* (1993) make the point that:

> *as the patient begins to relate his story, it is necessary to silence our own internal talk – that part of consciousness that is already forming the next comment, question, or criticism, even as the patient is still speaking, distracting our attention away from his experience and from our own spontaneous responses. The diagnostic reasoning process, too, is a kind of internal talk that can interfere with our ability to listen; it can safely be deferred for a few moments until the patient's story is completed.*

Haidet & Paterniti (2003) talk of 'mindful practice' as the ability of the physician to observe not only the patient during the medical interview, but himself as well.

Rapport

Matthews *et al.* (1993) suggest that the most basic element of connection is rapport, which depends on mutual respect and interest between clinician and patient.

Many patients have their own ideas of what has contributed to or caused their illness, and will want to tell the doctor. The doctor needs to be aware of these ideas in order to negotiate a mutual understanding which accommodates both views.

Mercer & Howie (2006) state that patients consistently rank empathy and humanness as a key attribute of a 'good doctor.'

Relationship

The Royal College of Physicians Report (2005) states that doctors aim to restore and strengthen both well-being and a patient's dignity:

> *Dignity emphasises ... the intrinsic moral worth of a human being and also the freedom and capacity – physical and mental – of the individual to live a life that they desire. Behaviours that strengthen trust include courtesy, kindness, understanding, humility, honesty, and confidentiality. These behaviours create an environment of safety around the patient.*

Frankel & Beckman (1989) report that 'patients were more satisfied if the doctor was warm (Francis *et al.* (1969), empathic (Wasserman *et al.*, 1984), and allowed the patient to share opinions during the interview (Stewart (1984).'

MacDonald (2004) reports: 'the consistent finding that physicians who adopt a warm, friendly and reassuring manner are more effective in therapeutic terms than those who keep consultations formal and do not offer reassurance.'

Emotional intelligence

Salovey & Mayer (1990) defined emotional intelligence (EI) as 'the ability to monitor one's own and others' feelings and emotions, to discriminate among them and to use this information to guide one's thinking and actions.' It focuses on how people appraise and communicate emotion, and how they use that emotion in solving problems and regulating behaviour.

The concept of EI was popularised by Goleman (1998) who defined an 'emotional competence' as a 'learned capability based on emotional intelligence that results in outstanding performance at work.'

However, there are two main reasons why we need to be cautious about embracing the idea of emotional intelligence *per se*. The first is that data are not available to confirm its value (Landy, 2005). Secondly, various researchers have argued that the definition of emotional intelligence has become too varied or all-encompassing to be useful (Locke, 2005).

Locke (2005) makes the following conclusion about emotional intelligence:

1. The definition of the concept is constantly changing.
2. Most definitions are so all-inclusive as to make the concept unintelligible.
3. One definition (eg reasoning with emotion) involves a contradiction.
4. There is no such thing as actual emotional intelligence, although intelligence can be applied to emotions as well as to other life domains.

Chapter 6: Models of the medical interview

The doctor, the patient and the context

It is clear that personal beliefs, attitudes, emotions or experiences in the past or in the present can influence the doctor's emotional response to patients: 'personal experiences in the doctor's life can determine professional actions' (Salinsky & Sackin, 2000).

McWhinney (1989) writes that:

All too frequently we do not listen to our patients, perceive their needs, or understand their sufferings. Understanding patients requires in the physician certain personal qualities not usually emphasised in medical education: self-knowledge, moral awareness, a reflective habit of mind, and a capacity for empathy and attentive listening.

The medical model

Levenstein *et al.* (1989) emphasise the distinction between the disease framework (What is the diagnosis?) and the illness framework (What is the patient's experience of illness: ideas, expectations and feelings?)

> Stewart & Roter (1989) explain that 'physicians bring to medical practice a world view based purely on the biomedical model, which emphasises biochemistry and technology. In contrast, a patient's world comprises a complex web of personality, culture, living situations, and relationships that colour and define the illness experience.'

Turner (2000) quotes several studies which report on the prevalence of affective disorder, which affects 13% of men and 17% of women admitted to general medical wards (Reid *et al.*, 2001); 20-25% of patients with diabetes or rheumatoid arthritis (Fink *et al.*, 1999); and over 30% of acute care admissions and patients with cancer (Hartz *et al.*, 2000).

The biopsychosocial model

> The biopsychosocial aspects of the patient-centred method include establishing a dialogue, understanding the meaning of the illness for the patient (McWhinney, 1989), and achieving a more humanistic interaction (Smith & Hoppe, 1991).

It makes sense that understanding a patient's thoughts and feelings about their illness will inform the doctor of how likely they are to follow advice or a certain treatment plan. Thoughts and perceptions influence actions.

> In terms of influencing or persuading, you have to know what a person believes and why they believe it before you can attempt to persuade them to do something else that you think would be better for them.

Ley (1998) explains that the health belief model states that the probability of an individual adopting a health conducive behaviour is affected by that individual's perceptions of:

- Their susceptibility to the illness or danger.
- The severity or seriousness of that illness or danger.
- The effectiveness or benefit of following the recommended course of action.
- The material and psychological costs of, and barriers to, the adoption of the behaviour.

Rollnick *et al.* (2005) state that:

> *When practitioners use a directing style, most of the consultation is taken up with informing patients about what the practitioner thinks they should do and why they should do it. When practitioners use a guiding style, they step aside from persuasion and instead encourage patients to explore their motivations and aspirations. The guiding style is more suited to consultations about changing behaviour because it harnesses the internal motivations of the patient. This was the starting point of motivational interviewing.*

Levinson *et al.* (2001) outline the stages of change model, which proposes that 'at a specific time, patients are in one of several discrete stages of change:

- Precontemplation;
- Contemplation;
- Determination;
- Action;
- Maintenance; or
- Relapse.

Typically, patients move from one stage to the next as they attempt to change. Relapse into the old unhealthy behavior (for example, smoking) is a common, almost expected, part of the change process.'

The psychodynamic model

In psychoanalysis, consideration of transference and countertransference is central to the analysis. Within the relationship between therapist and client, feelings arise toward each

> other that derive from past relationships. These feelings are projected onto the other person as though that person has 'caused' them, whereas in fact the person has simply triggered feelings from another time and place that were already there.

According to Freud (1997: 1910), 'transference arises spontaneously in all human relationships.'

> Countertransference is the doctor's emotional response to the patient.

Mollon (2001) points out that at least one third of consultations in primary care involve psychological problems.

The holistic model

> The Royal College of Physicians (2005) state that 'well-being indicates the holistic notion of achieving a state of health, comfort and happiness. It encompasses the physical, mental, and social aspects of a patient's life, aspects that the doctor seeks to heal or repair.'

The words health, healing and holistic all come from the same Germanic root, whole.

> Perez (2004): The spiritual aspects of medical care include: communication (listening, speaking), connection (space, safety, and sacredness), and communion through which healing can occur.'

Chapter 7: Barriers to communication

Racial and cultural differences

Tomorrow's Doctors (GMC, 2003) states that graduates must be able to do the following:

- Communicate effectively with individuals regardless of their social, cultural or ethnic backgrounds, or their disabilities.
- Communicate with individuals who cannot speak English, including working with interpreters.

> Good communication depends upon the ability to understand and be understood.

Schouten & Meeuwesen (2006) outlined five key predictors of culture-related communication problems which had been identified in the literature:

1. Cultural differences in explanatory models of health and illness;
2. Differences in cultural values;
3. Cultural differences in patients' preferences for doctor-patient, relationships;
4. Racism/perceptual biases;
5. Linguistic barriers.

> Many ethnic minority patients prefer to see a doctor of the same ethnic origin (Gray & Stoddard, 1997).

The important point is that every patient is an individual and even though they may belong to a particular racial or ethnic group, you cannot make assumptions about what that means to that individual.

> Coulehan *et al.* (2001) suggest guidelines for clinical empathy in the cross-cultural setting:
>
> - Understand your own cultural values and biases.
> - Develop a familiarity with the cultural values, health beliefs, and illness behaviours of ethnic, cultural, and religious groups served in your practice.
> - Ask how the patient prefers to be addressed.
> - Determine the patient's level of fluency in English and arrange for a translator, if needed.

- Assure the patient of confidentiality; rumours, jealousy, privacy, and reputation are crucial issues in close-knit traditional communities.
- Use a speech rate, tone, and style that promote understanding and show respect for the patient.
- Check back frequently to determine patient understanding and acceptance.

The balance of power

Goodyear-Smith & Buetow (2001) state that:

> *power is an inescapable aspect of all social relationships, and inherently is neither good nor evil. Doctors need power to fulfil their professional obligations to multiple constituencies including patients, the community and themselves. Patients need power to formulate their values, articulate and achieve health needs, and fulfil their responsibilities. However, both parties can use or misuse power.*

Bub (2006) states that 'illness and engagement with the healthcare system strip power away from the typical patient. The entire environment is unfamiliar, intimidating, and frightening, especially as patients are dependent on others for guidance and help.'

Various approaches to decision-making in medicine have been described, including the paternalistic, the shared and the informed approach.

The paternalistic approach involves eliciting physical symptoms and then the doctor making a diagnosis. 'In the "pure type" of this approach doctors can then make a treatment decision that they think is in their patients' best interest without having to explore each patient's values and concerns' (Charles *et al.*, 2000).

Charles *et al.* (2000) state that 'in the informed approach patients are accorded a more active role in both defining the problem for which they want help and in determining appropriate treatment. In the pure type of this approach the doctor's role is limited to providing relevant research information about treatment options and their benefits and risks so that the patient can make an informed decision.'

> In the shared approach, 'doctors commit themselves to an interactive relationship with patients in developing a treatment recommendation that is consistent with patient values and preferences' (Charles *et al.*, 2000).

Attitudes

MacDonald (2004) makes the point that 'some doctors just don't think that what patients have to say is of much interest.'

> Chochinov (2007) suggests a list of questions for doctors to ask themselves:
>
> • How would I be feeling in this patient's situation?
> • What is leading me to draw those conclusions?
> • Have I checked whether my assumptions are accurate?
> • Am I aware how my attitude towards the patient may be affecting him or her?
> • Could my attitude towards the patient be based on something to do with my own experiences, anxieties, or fears?
> • Does my attitude towards being a healthcare provider enable or disenable me to establish open and empathic professional relationships with my patients?

Chapter 8: Healing through relationship

The value of the holistic approach

Richards (1990) makes the point that 'even the briefest spell on the other side of the desk or in a hospital bed gives blinding insight into patients' vulnerability and of their need to be listened to, treated with respect, and given full, unhurried, jargon-free explanations. Simple gestures of kindness and encouragement go a long way – as does the occasional admission of fallibility.'

Salinsky & Sackin (2000) reported how becoming more aware of their own feelings made doctors more aware of the feelings that their patients were experiencing and trying to communicate to them.

Salinsky & Sackin (2000) state that: 'if our defences are too rigid, if we are unable to take a few risks with our feelings, then we find ourselves professionally disabled in a different way. To give an obvious example, we may miss a diagnosis of depression.' It has been pointed out that 'depression is among the most common conditions in primary care patients, yet studies find that physicians do not adequately detect or treat 40% to 60% of cases' (Center *et al..*, 2003).

Haidet & Paterniti (2003) encourage us towards mindful practice: 'the ability of the physician to observe not only the patient during the medical interview, but himself/herself as well.' In this way, learning about ourselves informs our interaction with others.

Being authentic in the moment
* Being authentic means bringing the whole of yourself to your interactions with patients – being genuine, spontaneous, thinking and feeling. Patients can see if we are defensive, closed down, inaccessible.
* Being flexible. Be prepared to try different approaches – if one doesn't work, then try another.
* You cannot be formulaic. What works for one person will often not work for another. Each patient is different; everyone wants to feel unique, important and individual.
* Communication is about relationship – you have to connect before you can truly communicate.
* Remembering Confucius: 'Never impose on others what you would not choose for yourself.'

Chapter 9: Life and death

Introduction to breaking bad news

Garg *et al.* (1997) state that 'breaking bad news is one of the most difficult tasks a physician or any other member of the health care team has to do. The way it is done may change the nature of the relationship permanently – strengthening it, undermining it, damaging it irreparably or even leading to litigation.'

The BMA (2004) quote Buckman (1984) who defines bad news as 'information likely to alter drastically a patient's view of his or her future.'

Girgis & Sanson-Fisher (1995) outline a summary of principles for breaking bad news:

1. One person only should be responsible for breaking bad news.
2. The patient has a legal and moral right to information.
3. Primary responsibility is to the individual patient.
4. Give accurate and reliable information.
5. Ask people how much they want to know.
6. Prepare the patient for the possibility of bad news as early as possible.
7. Avoid giving the results of each test individually, if several tests are being performed.
8. Tell the patient his/her diagnosis as soon as it is certain.
9. Ensure privacy and make the patient feel comfortable.
10. Ideally, family and significant others should be present.
11. If possible, arrange for another health professional to be present.
12. Inform the patient's general practitioner and other medical advisers of level of development of patient's understanding.
13. Use eye contact and body language to convey warmth, sympathy, encouragement, or reassurance to the patient.
14. Employ a trained health interpreter if language differences exist.

> 15. Be sensitive to the person's culture, race, religious beliefs, and social background.
> 16. Acknowledge your own shortcomings and emotional difficulties in breaking bad news.

Travaline *et al.* (2005) detail a list of practical steps:

1. Assess what the patient already knows about his or her condition to prevent confusion when new information is introduced.
2. Assess what the patient wants to know: not all patients with the same diagnosis want the same level of detail in the information offered about their condition or treatment.
3. Be empathic: recognize, acknowledge and explore the indirectly expressed emotions of patients.
4. Slow down: provide information in a slow and deliberate fashion, pause frequently.
5. Keep it simple: short statements and clear, simple explanations.
6. Tell the truth
7. Be hopeful: being able to promise comfort and minimal suffering has real value.
8. Watch the patient's body and face: facial expressions are often good indicators of sadness, worry, or anxiety.
9. Be prepared for a reaction: give sufficient time for a full display of emotions, listen quietly and attentively to what the patient or family are saying.

How to break bad news – some practical advice

- The first thing to decide is the degree of urgency in telling the bad news.
- In preparing for the discussion, make sure you have all the facts before giving the news.
- Before going to see the patient or relatives, it is a good idea to give yourself time to calm yourself, and to think about how you are going to start the conversation.
- Find the right place to give the news. It needs to be private and you need to have enough time to talk it through.
- It is good practice to try and get rid of your bleep and phone for the duration of the interview.

- It is best to write in the notes after the conversation.
- Determine what patients know already and how much information they want.
- Determine whether to tell a patient alone or with relatives.
- There are a few golden rules in giving news: don't lie, don't use jargon, don't use euphemisms. And listen to the patient.
- The important thing is to have a conversation. Show empathy, allow silences.
- Give the patient time to take in the news you have just given them.
- Remember it is always very difficult to try to predict how long a person has to live.
- Ask the patient or relative whether they have any questions and reassure them that they can come back in the future if they think of things that they would like to ask.

The process of breaking bad news and caring for people as they adjust to that news can be very rewarding. It is a hugely important event for that person, and it's vital to take the time to learn how to do it well. They are likely to remember it forever.

End-of-life care

In the United Kingdom almost a quarter of occupied hospital bed days are taken up by patients who are in the last year of life, and some 60% of all deaths occur there (Clark, 2005).

The term 'palliative care' was first proposed in 1974 by the Canadian surgeon, Balfour Mount (Clark, 2005). The World Health Organisation defines it as 'the active total care of patients whose disease is not responsive to curative treatment. Control of pain, of other symptoms and of psychological, social and spiritual problems is paramount. The goal of palliative care is achievement of the best possible quality of life for patients and their families' (Saunders, 1996).

Buckman (2002) makes the point that 'communication is often a major component of the medical management in chronic and palliative care: sometimes it is all we have to offer.'

The Royal College of Physicians (1997) state that:

> *Doctors become anxious about giving bad news because they fear that patients will become distressed, emotionally disorganised, ask difficult or impossible questions, express disappointment, blame or anger and will find it unusually difficult to see the clinical facts in perspective. Doctors also fear being in a position of not knowing all the answers, the loss of the familiar support of clinical authority and loss of control. They may also be aware that they do not have the skill to comfort distressed patients and relatives and also that to do so threatens to be time-consuming.*

If psychological issues are not explored, important problems can be overlooked. Newell *et al.* (1998) report that only 17% of patients classified as clinically anxious and 6% of those classified as clinically depressed were perceived as such by their oncologists.

Chapter 10: Dealing with difficult situations

Managing conflict in the team

In their report on medical professionalism, the Royal College of Physicians (2005) stated that 'The keys to strong clinical teams are recognition, mutual respect, and an appreciation of the constant redefinition of boundaries among the team.'

With the recent introduction of the European Working Time Directive, 'the increasing use of shift systems for junior doctors can lead to a further splintering of care, making the introduction of safe methods of communication at hand-over times essential' (RCP, 1997).

The Medical Leadership Competency Framework drawn up by the Academy of Medical Royal Colleges and the Institute for Innovation and Improvement (2005) states that in order to be able to work within teams, doctors must:

- Have a clear sense of their role, responsibilities and purpose within the team.

- Adopt a team approach, acknowledging and appreciating efforts, contributions and compromises.
- Recognise the common purpose of the team and respect team decisions.
- Listen to others.
- Empathise and take into account the needs and feelings of others.
- Communicate effectively with individuals and groups.
- Gain and maintain the trust and support of colleagues.

The Framework states that in working with others, doctors should:

- Provide encouragement and opportunity for people to engage in decision-making.
- Respect, value and acknowledge the roles, contributions and expertise of others.
- Employ strategies to manage conflict of interests and differences of opinion.
- Keep the focus of contribution on delivering and improving services to patients.

Handling difficult patients

Most doctors felt that their own reasons for perceiving patients as difficult were: workload, lack of job satisfaction, their own psychic condition, and lack of training in counselling and communication skills (Serour *et al.*, 2009).

Levinson *et al.* (1993) found that of doctors in busy practice settings, '36% reported frustration in 11–25% of visits. 8% felt frustrated in up to half of their patient encounters. The cause of the frustrating visits was most frequently attributed to the nature of the patient.'

Butler *et al.* (1999) suggest ways to manage the heartsink patient, including:

- Improving clinicians' self-awareness, counselling, and consultation skills.

- The doctor provides the patient with the opportunity to communicate, which can result in brief, intense, and close contact that can be deeply therapeutic.
- The 'holding strategy' whereby positive attempts to bring about change are abandoned in favour of simply listening to the patient without contradicting him/her.
- Improving doctors' working conditions to reduce stress and enable them to cope better with difficult situations.
- Enhancing understanding and sharing responsibility through team discussion.

Managing aggression and violence

Perrin (1997) reports that 'it has been estimated that 50% of health care staff will be physically assaulted at least once at some point in their careers.'

The National Institute for Health and Clinical Excellence's (NICE, 2005) guidelines *The Short-Term Management of Disturbed/ Violent Behaviour in In-Patient Psychiatric Setting and Emergency Department*:

- De-escalation involves the use of techniques that calm down an escalating situation or service user; therefore, action plans should stress that de-escalation should be employed early on in any escalating situation.
- A service user's anger needs to be treated with an appropriate, measured and reasonable response.
- Staff should accept that in a crisis situation they are responsible for avoiding provocation. It is not realistic to expect the person exhibiting disturbed/violent behaviour to simply calm down.
- Staff should learn to recognise what generally and specifically upsets and calms people. This will involve listening to individual service users and carer's reports of what upsets the service user, and this should be reflected in the service user's care plan.
- Staff should be aware of, and learn to monitor and control, their own verbal and non-verbal behaviour, such as body posture and eye contact.

- Where possible and appropriate, service users should be encouraged to recognise their own trigger factors, early warning signs of disturbed/violent behaviour, and other vulnerabilities. This information should be included in care plans and a copy given to the service user. Service users should also be encouraged to discuss and negotiate their wishes should they become agitated.
- Where de-escalation techniques fail to sufficiently calm a situation or service user, staff should remember that verbal de-escalation is an ongoing element of the management of an escalating individual. Verbal de-escalation is supported but not replaced by appropriate physical intervention.

Patients with mental health problems

Even if a person is depressed, psychotic, or intent on self-destruction, there is often a part, albeit small, that wants to keep safe and get better. If you can enlist the help of this part then you can start a dialogue.

Maguire (2000) states that 'most withdrawn patients will acknowledge that they are indeed finding it difficult to get into conversation.' He suggests a number of ways of drawing the patient out:

'I get the feeling that we are finding it difficult to get into a discussion about your problems.'
'I have to work with the part of you that is willing to try and confront your problems so that I can see if we can do anything about them.'

Complaints

Dyer (2009) states that 'the number of doctors complained about to the General Medical Council rose by 32% between 2002 and 2008, from 4452 doctors in 2002 to 5195 in 2008.'

The Royal College of Physicians (1997) state that 'feelings of regretful sympathy for suffering can and should be expressed even where a complaint may be unjustified or where no one is at fault. A doctor who says that he or she is sorry that a patient has suffered is not admitting liability and should not fear possible litigation in simply expressing sympathy or regret.'

MacDonald (2004) reports that 'when mistakes have been made patients need to know the exact nature and scale of the error. They need to know the possible implications and long-term effects of such a mistake. They need to know how it came about that the mistake was made and what steps have been put in place to prevent the same error occurring again.'

Chapter 11: New directions

Looking after ourselves

De Mercato *et al.* (1995) assessed the prevalence of the burnout syndrome in physicians, nurses, and ancillary medical workers, and found that, overall, 45.5% reported symptoms of burnout.

McManus *et al.* (2002) conducted a three-year longitudinal study of 331 UK doctors in which they assessed stress and the three components of burnout (emotional exhaustion, depersonalization, and low personal accomplishment). They found that 'emotional exhaustion and stress showed reciprocal causation: high levels of emotional exhaustion caused stress, and high levels of stress caused emotional exhaustion.

Maguire (2000) makes the point that 'doctors appear to be more at risk of burnout if they believe that denial of their own personal needs is desirable or that their own uncertainties and emotions must be kept private.'

Turner (2001) makes the point that 'clinicians may be exhausted by the emotional needs of their patients … they cannot provide excellent clinical care if they fail to nurture themselves physically, emotionally and spiritually.'

Support and supervision

Novack *et al.* (1997) suggest 'organized activities that can promote physician personal awareness such as support groups, Balint groups, and discussions of meaningful experiences in medicine. Experience with these activities suggests that through enhancing personal awareness physicians can improve their clinical care and increase satisfaction with work, relationships, and themselves.'

Reflection

Bishop (2002) explains that 'Mindfulness-Based Stress Reduction (MBSR) is a clinical program, developed to facilitate adaptation to medical illness, which provides systematic training in mindfulness meditation as a self-regulatory approach to stress reduction and emotion management. There has been widespread and growing use of this approach within medical settings in the last twenty years.'

Chiesa & Serretti (2009) state that 'MBSR is able to reduce stress levels in healthy people.

Praissman (2008) conducted a literature review which showed that 'both patients and healthcare providers experiencing stress or stress-related symptoms benefit from MBSR programs. They concluded that MBSR is a safe, effective, integrative approach for reducing stress, and that it is therapeutic for healthcare providers, enhancing their interactions with patients.'

Intuitively, it makes sense that when we can look after ourselves, then we are better able to look after others.

List of abbreviations

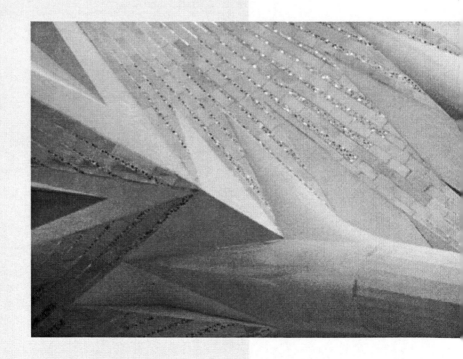

List of abbreviations

BMA	British Medical Association
BMJ	British Medical Journal
DH	Department of Health
EEA	European Economic Area
EI	Emotional Intelligence
MBTI	Myers-Brigg Type Indicator
MRCGP	Membership of the Royal College of General Practitioners
MBSR	Mindfulness-Based Stress Reduction
NHS	National Health Service
NICE	National Institute for Health and Clinical Excellence
PMETB	Postgraduate Medical Education and Training Board
QAA	Quality Assurance Agency
RCP	Royal College of Practitioners
RCS	Royal College of Surgeons
RPS	Royal Pharmaceutical Society
WAIS	Wechsler Adult Intelligence Scale
WHO	World Health Organisation
WMA	World Medical Association

References

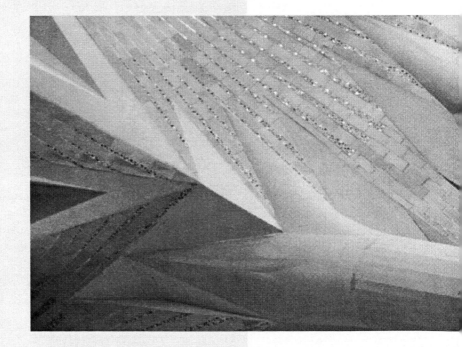

References

Abramovitch, H., & Schwartz., E. (1996) Three stages of medical dialogue. *Theoretical Medicine*: 17: 175–187

Ahlén, G.C., Mattsson, B., and Gunnarsson, R.K. (2007) Physician–patient questionnaire to assess physician–patient agreement at the consultation. *Family Practice*: 24(5):498–503

Agerbo, E., Gunnell, D., Bonde, J.P., Mortensen, P.B., and Nordentoft, M. (2007) Suicide and occupation: the impact of socio-economic, demographic and psychiatric differences. *Psychological Medicine*: 37(8): 1131–1140.

Ahmed-Little, Y. (2009) The European Working Time Directive 2009. *Br J Health Care Manag*: 12: 373–6.

Ahrens, T., Yancey, V., and Kollef, M. (2003) Improving Family Communications at the End of Life: Implications for Length of Stay in the Intensive Care Unit and Resource Use. *American Journal of Critical Care*: 12: 317–324

Ambuel, B., Butler, D., Hamberger, L.K., Lawrence, S., and Guse, C.E. (2003) Female and male medical students' exposure to violence: impact on well being and perceived capacity to help battered women. *J Comp Fam Stud*: 34: 113–35.

Anonymous. (1994) Burnished or burnt out: The delights and dangers of working in health. *The Lancet*: 344: 1583–1584.

Arora, N.K., & McHorney, C.A. (2000) Patient preference for medical decision making: Who really wants to participate? *Medical Care*: 38: 335–341.

Aspegren, K. (1999) BEME guide no 2: Teaching and learning communication skills in medicine – a review with quality grading of articles. *Medical Teacher*: 21: 563–570.

Awalt, R.M., Reilly, P.M., and Shopshire, M.S. (1997) The angry patient: An intervention for managing anger in substance abuse treatment. *Journal of Psychoactive Drugs*: 29: 353–358.

Baile, W.F., Kudelka, A.P., Beale, E.A., Glober, G.A., Myers, E.G., Greisinger, A.J., and Bast, R.C. Jr. (1999) Communication skills training in oncology. Description and preliminary outcomes of workshops on breaking bad news and managing patient reactions to illness. *Cancer Nurse*: 86: 887–897.

Balint, M. (1957) *The doctor, his patient and the illness*. London, Churchill Livingstone.

Barnett, P.B. (2001) Rapport and the hospitalist. *Am J Med*: 111: 31S–35S

Bar-On, R. & Parker, J.D.A. (2000) *Handbook of Emotional Intelligence*. San Francisco, Jossey-Bass,.

Barry, C.A., Bradley, C.P., Britten, N., Stevenson, F.A., and Barber, N. (2000) Patients' unvoiced agendas in general practice consultations: qualitative study. *BMJ*: 320:1246–1250.

Barsky, A.J. 3rd. (1981) Hidden reasons some patients visit doctors. *Annals of Internal Medicine*: 94: 492–8,

Barzansky, B., Jonas, H.S., and Etzel, S.I. (2000) Educational Programs in US Medical Schools, 1999–2000. *JAMA*: 284(9):1114–1120

Batenburg, V., Smal, J.A., Lodder, A., and de Melker, R.A. (1999) Are professional attitudes related to gender and medical specialty? *Medical Education*: 33: 489–492

Beach, M.C., Roter, D., Rubin, H., Frankel, R., Levinson, W., and Ford, D.E. (2004) Is Physician Self-disclosure Related to Patient Evaluation of Office Visits? *J Gen Intern Med*: 19: 905–910.

Beach, M.C., Sugarman, J., Johnson, R.L., Arbelaez, J.J., Duggan, P.S., and Cooper, L.A. (2005) Do patients treated with dignity report higher satisfaction, adherence and receipt of preventive care. *Ann Fam Med*: 3:331–338.

Beach, M.C., Roter, D.L., Wang, N.Y., Duggan, P.S., and Cooper, L,A. (2006) Are physicians' attitudes of respect accurately perceived by patients and associated with more positive communication behaviors? *Patient Education & Counseling*: 62(3):347–354

Beckman, H.B., & Frankel, R.M. (1984) The effect of physician behaviour on the collection of data. *Ann Intern Med*: 101: 692–696.

References

Beckman, H.B., Frankel, R.M., and Delaney, J. (1985) Soliciting the patients complete agenda: A relationship to the distribution of concerns. *Clinical Research*: 33: 714A.

Beckman, H., Kaplan, S.H., Frankel, R. (1989) Outcome based research on doctor-patient communication: A review. In: Stewart, M., & Roter, D. editors, *Communicating with Medical Patients*, Beverley Hills, CA, Sage publications, pp 223–227

Bellini, L.M., Baime, M., and Shea, J.A. (2002) Variation of mood and empathy during internship. *JAMA*: 287: 3143–3146

Berger, J.T., Coulehan, J., and Belling, C. (2004) Humor in the physician-patient encounter. *Arch Intern Med*: 164: 825–830

Berry, D. (2007) *Health Communication: Theory and Practice*. Maidenhead, Open University Press.

Bertakis, K.D. (1977) The communication of information from physician to patient: a method for increasing patient retention and satisfaction. *J Fam Pract*: 5: 217–222

Betz Brown, J., Boles, M., Mulloly, J.P., and Levinson, W. (1999) Effect of clinician communication skills training on patient satisfaction. *Annals of Internal Medicine*: 131: 822–829.

Bishop, S.R. (2002) What do we really know about Mindfulness-Based Stress Reduction? *Psychosomatic Medicine*: 64: 71–83.

Blum, L.H. (1985) Beyond medicine: Healing power in the doctor-patient relationship. *Psychological Reports*: 57: 399–427.

Bonner, G., & McLaughlin, S. (2007) The psychological impact of aggression on nursing staff. *British Journal of Nursing*: 16: 810–4.

Boyatzis, R.E., Goleman, D., and Rhee, K.S. (2000) Clustering competence in emotional intelligence: Insights from the emotional competence inventory. In Bar-On, R., & Parker, J.D.A. *The Handbook of Emotional Intelligence*. San Francisco, Jossey-Bass.

Boyle, G.J., Matthew, G., and Saklofske, D.H. (2008) *Personality theory and assessment. Personality measurement and testing*. London, Sage Publications.

Branch, W.T. Jr. (2006) Viewpoint: Teaching Respect for Patients. *Academic Medicine*: 81: 463–467

Bristol Royal Infirmary Inquiry. (2001) *Learning from Bristol: the report of the public inquiry into children's heart surgery at the Bristol Royal Infirmary 19841995*. London, HMSO.

British Medical Association. (2004) *Communication education skills for doctors: an update*. London, British Medical Association.

Britten, N., Ukoumunne, O.C., and Boulton, M.G. (2002) Patients' attitudes to medicines and expectations for prescriptions. *Health Expect*: 5: 256–269.

Brody, D.S., Miller, S.M., Lerman, C.E., Smith, D.G., and Caputo, G.C. (1989) Patient perception of involvement in medical care: relationship to illness attitudes and outcomes. *Journal of General Internal Medicine*: 4(6): 506–11.

Bruijnzeels, M., & Visser, A. (2005) Intercultural doctor-patient relational outcomes: Need more to be studied. *Patient Education and Counseling*: 57: 151–152.

Bub, B. (2006) *Communication Skills that Heal: a practical approach to a new professionalism in medicine*. Oxford, Radcliffe Publishing.

Buckman, R. (1984) Breaking bad news: why is it still so difficult? *BMJ*: 288: 1597–9.

Buckman, R. (2002) Communications and emotions: Skills and effort are the key. *BMJ*: 325: 672

Bull, P. (2001) State of the art: Nonverbal communication. *Psychologist*: 14, 12: 644.

Burack, R.C., & Carpenter, R.R. (1983) The predictive value of the presenting complaint. *J Fam Pract*: 16: 749–54.

Bury, M. (2001) Illness narratives: fact or fiction? *Sociology of Health & Illness*: 23: 263–285.

Butler, C.C., & Evans, M., and The Welsh Philosophy and General Practice discussion Group (1999) The 'heartsink' patient revisited. *British Journal of General Practice*: 49(440): 230–3.

References

Butow, P.N., Brown, R.F., Cogar, S., Tattersall, M.H., and Dunn, S.M. (2002) Oncologist´s reactions to cancer patients´ verbal cues. *Psycho-oncology*: 11: 47–58.

Buyck, D., & Lang, F. (2002) Teaching medical communications skills: a call for greater uniformity. *Fam Med*: 34(5): 337–343.

Byrne, P.S., & Long, B.E.L. (1976) *Doctors talking to patients*. HMSO, London.

Calkins, D.R., Rubenstein, L.V., Cleary, P.D., Davies, A.R., Jette, A.M., Fink, A., Kosecoff, J., Young, R.T., Brook, R.H., and Delbanco, T.L. *et al.*: (1991) Failure of physicians to recognize functional disability in ambulatory patients. *Ann Intern Med* 114: 451–454.

Campion, P.D., Butler, N.M., and Cox, A.D. (1992) Principal agendas of doctors and patients in research and practice. *J Med Educ*: 54: 498–500

Campion, P., Foulkes, J., Neighbour, R., and Tate, P. (2002) Patient-centeredness in the MRCGP video examination: analysis of large cohort. *BMJ*: 325: 691–2.

Cairns, H., Hendry, B., Leather, A., and Moxham, J. (2008) Outcomes of the European Working Time Directive. *BMJ*: 337: a942.

Call to tackle burnout among medics. *BMA News*, November 14, 2009, pp4.

Carmody, J., & Baer, R.A. (2008) Relationships between mindfulness practice and levels of mindfulness, medical and psychological symptoms and well-being in a mindfulness-based stress reduction program. *Journal of Behavioral Medicine*: 31: 23–33.

Carotenuto, A., & Tambureno, J. (1991) *Kant's dove: The history of transference in psychoanalysis*: New York, Chiron publications.

Carroll B.T., Kathol, R.G., Noyes, R., Wald, T.G., and Clamon, G.H. (1993) Screening for depression and anxiety in cancer patients using the hospital anxiety and depression scale. *Gen Hosp Psychiatry*: 15: 69 –74.

Castledine, S.G. (2008) Dealing with difficult doctors. *British Journal of Nursing*: 17: 1305

Cegala, D.J., & Broz, S.L. (2002) Physician communication skills training: a review of theoretical backgrounds, objectives and skills. *Med Edu*: 36: 1004–1016.

Center, C., Davis, M., Detre, T., Ford, D.E., Hansbrough, W., Hendin, H., Laszlo, J., Litts, D.A., Mann, J., Mansky, P.A., Michels, R., Miles, S.H., Proujansky, R., Reynolds, C.F., and Silverman, M.M. (2003) Confronting depression and suicide in physicians: a consensus statement. *JAMA*: 289: 3161–6.

Centre for Change and Innovation. (2003) *Talking matters: Developing the communication skills of doctors*. Edinburgh, Scottish Executive.

Charles, C., Gafni, A., and Whelan, T. (2000) How to improve communication between doctors and patients. *BMJ*: 320: 1220–1221.

Charon, R. (2001) Narrative medicine: A model for empathy, reflection, profession and trust. *JAMA*: 286(15): 1897–1902.

Chiesa, A., & Serretti, A. (2009) Mindfulness-based stress reduction for stress management in healthy people: a review and meta-analysis. *Journal of Alternative & Complementary Medicine*: 15: 593–600.

Chochinov, H.M. (2007) Dignity and the essence of medicine: the A, B, C, and D of dignity conserving care. *BMJ*: 335: 184–7.

Clack, G.B., Allen, J., Cooper, D., and O Head, J. (2004) Personality differences between doctors and their patients: implications for the teaching of communication skills. *Medical Education*: 38: 177–86.

Clark, D. (2002) Between hope and acceptance: the medicalisation of dying. *BMJ*: 324: 905–907

Clark, D. (2005) *Cicely Saunders – Founder of the Hospice Movement: Selected Letters* 1959–1999. Oxford, Oxford University Press.

Clark, J., & Armit, K. (2008) Attainment of competency in management and leadership: No longer an optional extra for doctors. *Clinical Governance*: 13: 35–42.

Cockburn, J., & Pit, S. (1997) Prescribing behaviour in clinical practice: patients' expectations and doctors perception of patients expectations. *BMJ*: 315: 520–523.

References

Cohen, D., Rollnick, S., Smail, S., Kinnersley, P., Houston, H., and Edwards, K. (2005) Communication, stress and distress: evolution of an individual support programme for medical students and doctors. *Medical Education*: 36(5): 476–481.

Colletti, L., Gruppen, L., Barclay, M., and Stern, D. (2001) Teaching students to break bad news. *Am J Surg*: 182: 20–23.

Confederation of British Industry (2005) *Who cares wins: The benefits of positive absence management*. London, Confederation of British Industry.

Coombs, M. (2003) Power and conflict in intensive care clinical decision making. *Intensive and Critical Care Nursing*: 19: 125–135.

Coombs, M., & Ersser, S.J. (2004) Medical hegemony in decision-making – a barrier to interdisciplinary working in intensive care? *Journal of Advanced Nursing*: 46: 245–252.

Cork, A., & Ferns, T. (2008) Managing alcohol related aggression in the emergency department (Part II). *International Emergency Nursing*: 16: 88–93.

Corradi, R.B. (2006) A conceptual model of transference and its psychotherapeutic application. *Journal of the American Academy of Psychoanalysis and Dynamic Psychiatry*: 34(3): 415–439.

Costa, P.T.Jr., & McCrae, R.R. (1992). *Revised NEO Personality Inventory (NEO-PI-R) and NEO Five-Factor Inventory (NEO-FFI) manual*. Odessa, FL, Psychological Assessment Resources.

Coulehan, J.L., Platt, F.W., Egener, B., Frankel, R., Lin, C.T., Lown, B., and Salazar, W.H. (2001) "Let me see if I have this right....": Words that help build empathy. *Annals of Internal Medicine*: 135: 221–226.

Coulter, A. (1999) Paternalism or partnership? Patients have grown up – and there's no going back. *BMJ*: 319: 719–720.

Coulter, A., Entwistle, V., and Gilbert, D. (1999) Sharing decisions with patients: is the information good enough? *BMJ*: 318: 318–322.

Coulter, A. (2002a) After Bristol: putting patients at the centre. *BMJ*: 324: 648–51

Coulter, A. (2002b) Patients views of the good doctor. *BMJ*: 325: 668–669

Cox, A., Hopkinson, K., and Rutter, M. (1981) Psychiatric interviewing techniques. II. Naturalistic study. *Br J Psychiatry*: 138: 283–291.

Cox, A. (1989) Eliciting patients' feelings. In: Stewart, M., & Roter, D. editors, *Communicating with Medical Patients*, Beverley Hills, CA, Sage Publications, pp 99–106

Cumming, A. (2002) Good communication skills can mask deficiencies. *BMJ*: 325: 676.

Davis, M.A., Hoffman, J.R., and Hsu, J. (1999) Impact of patient acuity on preference for information and autonomy in decision making. *Acad Emerg Med*: 6: 781–785

Professor the Lord Darzi of Denham KBE (2008) *High quality care for all: NHS Next Stage Review final report*. London, HMSO.

Davies, S. (2001) Assaults and threats on psychiatrists. *Psychiatric Bulletin*: 25(3): 89–91.

Day, M. The rise of the doctor-manager. *BMJ*, 2007: 335: 230–231.

Deber, R. (1994) The patient-physician partnership: changing roles and the desire for information. *Can Med Assoc J*: 151: 171–176.

Degner, L.F., & Sloan, J.A. (1992) Decision making during serious illness: what role to patients really want to play? *J Clin Epidemiol*: 45: 941–950.

DeLahunta, E., & Tulsky, A. (1996) Personal exposure of faculty and medical students to family violence. *JAMA*: 275: 1903–6.

Delaney, G. (2007) A farewell to heart sink? *British Journal of General Practice*: 57: 584–585

Delbanco, T., & Sands, D.Z. (2004) Electrons in flight – e-mail between doctors and patients. *NEJM*: 350: 1705–1707.

de Mercato, R., Cantiello, G., Celentano, U., Romano, A., *et al.*. (1995) Burnout syndrome in medical and non medical staff: Preliminary results. *New Trends in Experimental & Clinical Psychiatry*: 11: 43–45.

Department of Health. (2001a) *Working together, learning together: a framework for lifelong learning*. London, HMSO.

References

Department of Health. (2001b) *The expert patient: A new approach to chronic disease management for the 21st century*. London, HMSO

Department of Health. (2006) White paper – *Our health, our care, our say: a new direction for community services*. London, HMSO.

Department of Health. (2007) White paper – *Trust, Assurance and safety: The regulation of health professionals*. London, HMSO.

Department of Health. (2009) *The NHS Constitution for England*. London, HMSO.

DiMatteo, M.R., & Taranta, A. (1979) Nonverbal Communication and Physician/Patient Rapport: An Empirical Study. Professional *Psychology: August*: 540–547

DiMatteo, M.R., Taranta, A., Friedman, H.S., and Prince, L.M. (1980) Predicting patient satisfaction from physicians'nonverbal communication skill. *Med Care*: 18: 376–387.

DiMatteo, M.R., Hays, R.D., and Prince, L.M. (1986) Relationship of physicians' nonverbal communication skill to patient satisfaction, appointment noncompliance, and physician workload. *Health Psychology*: 5(6): 581–594.

DiMatteo, R., & Chow, M.S.S. (1995) Patient adherence to pharmacotherapy: The importance of effective communication. *Formulary*: 30: 596–605.

DiMatteo, M.R., Lepper, H.S, and Croghan, T.W. (2000) Depression is a risk factor for non-compliance with medical treatment: Meta-analysis of the effects of anxiety and depression on patient adherence. *Arch Intern Med*: 160: 2101–2107.

DiMatteo, M.R. (2004a) Variations in patients' adherence to medical recommendations: a quantitative review of 50 years of research. *Medical Care*: 42(3): 200–209.

DiMatteo, M.R. (2004b) Social support and patient adherence to medical treatment: a meta-analysis. *Health Psychology*: 23(2): 207–218.

DiMatteo, M.R., Haskard, M.R., and Williams, S.L. (2007) Health beliefs, disease severity, and patient adherence: a meta-analysis. *Medical care*: 45(6): 521–528.

Disiker, R., & Michiellute, A. (1981) An analysis of empathy in medical students before and following clinical experience. *Journal of Medical Education*: 56: 1004–1010.

Dixon, D.M., Sweeney, K.G., and Pereira Gray, D.J. (1999) The physician healer: Ancient magic or modern science? *British Journal of General Practice*: 49: 309–312

Dosanjh, S., Barnes, J., and Bhandari, M. (2001) Barriers to breaking bad news among medical and surgical residents. *Medical Education*: 35: 197–205.

Dowell, J., Jones, A., and Snadden, D. (2002) Exploring medication use to seek concordance with ´non-adherent´ patients: a qualitative study. *British Journal of General Practice*: 52: 24–32.

Dunn, S.M., Butow, P.N., Tattersall, M.H., Jones, Q.J., Sheldon, J.S., Taylor, J.J., and Sumich, M.D. (1993) General information tapes inhibit recall of the cancer consultation. *Journal of Clinical Oncology*: 11: 2279–2285.

Dyer, C. (2009) Rate of serious complaints against UK doctors is higher for those qualifying outside Europe. *BMJ*: 338: 1983.

Edwards, A. (2003) Communicating risks. *BMJ*: 327: 691–2.

Edwards, N., Kornacki, M.J., and Silversin, J. (2002) Unhappy doctors: what are the causes and what can be done? *BMJ*: 324: 835–838.

Egnew, T.R. (2009) Suffering, meaning, and healing: challenges of contemporary medicine. *Annals of Family Medicine*: 7(2): 170–5

Eisenthal, S., & Lazare, A. (1976) Evaluation of the initial interview in a walk-in clinic. The patient's perspective on a "customer approach". *Journal of Nervous & Mental Disease*: 162(3): 169–176.

Eisenthal, S., Emery, R., Lazare, A., and Udin, H. (1979) "Adherence" and the negotiated approach to patienthood. *Archives of General Psychiatry*: 36: 393–398.

Elwyn, G., Edwards, A., Mowle, S., Wensing, M., Wildinson, C., Kinnersley, P., and Grol, R. (2001) Measuring the involvement of patients in shared decision making: a systematic review of instruments. *Patient Educ Couns*: 43: 5–22.

References

Elwyn, G., Edwards, A., Britten, N. (2003) 'Doing prescribing': how doctors can be more effective. *BMJ*: 327: 864–867.

Engel, G.L. (1997) From Biomedical to Biopsychosocial: Being Scientific in the Human Domain. *Psychosomatics*: 38: 521–528.

Engel, P.A. (2001) George L. Engel, M.D., 1913–1999: Remembering His Life and Works; Rediscovering His Soul. *Psychosomatics*: 42: 94–99.

Epel, E., Daubenmier, J., Moskowitz, J.T., Folkman, S., and Blackburn, E. (2009) Can meditation slow rate of cellular aging? Cognitive stress, mindfulness, and telomeres. *Annals of the New York Academy of Sciences*: 1172: 34–53.

Evans, B.J., Stanley, R.O., Mestrovic, R., and Rose, L. (1991) Effects of communication skills training on students' diagnostic efficiency. *Medical Education*: 25: 517–526.

Faden, R.R., Becker, C., Lewis, C., Freeman, J., and Faden, A.I. (1981) Disclosure of information to patients in medical care. *Medical Care*: 19(7): 718–33

Fallowfield, L.J., Maguire, G.P., and Baum, M. (1990) Psychological outcomes of different treatment policies in women with early breast cancer outside a clinical trial. *BMJ*: 301: 575–580.

Fallowfield, L.J., Hall, A., Maguire, P., Baum, M., and A'Hern, R.P. (1994) Psychological effects of being offered choice of surgery for breast cancer. *BMJ*: 309: 448.

Fallowfield, L., & Jenkins, V. (1999) Effective communication skills are the key to good cancer care. *Eur J Canc*: 35(11): 1592–7.

Fallowfield, L., Jenkins, V., Farewell, V., Saul, J., Duffy, A., and Eves, R. (2002) Efficacy of a Cancer Research UK communication skills training model for oncologists: a randomised controlled trial. *The Lancet*: 359: 9307.

Feinmann, J. (2002) Brushing up on doctors' communication skills. *The Lancet*: 360:1572.

Ferguson, W.J., & Candib, L.M. (2002) Culture, language and the doctor–patient relationship. *Fam Med*: 34: 353–361.

Ferner, R.E. (2002) Is concordance the primrose path to health? *BMJ*: 327: 821–822.

Forster, H.P., Schwartz, J., and DeRenzo, E. (2002) Reducing legal risk by practicing patient-centered medicine. *Arch Intern Med*: 162: 1217–1219.

Forster, J.A., Petty, M.T., Schleiger, C., and Walters, H.C. (2005) Know workplace violence: Developing programs for managing the risk of aggression in the health care setting. *Medical Journal of Australia*: 183: 357–361.

Foster T. (2003) Suicide note themes and suicide prevention. Int J Psychiatry Med: 33: 323–31.

Frankel, R., & Beckman, H. (1989) Evaluating the patient's primary problem(s). In: Stewart, M., & Roter, D. editors, *Communicating with Medical Patients*, Beverley Hills, CA, Sage Publications, pp 86–98

Freeman, G.K., Horder, J.P., Howie, J.G.R., Hungin, A.P., Hill, A.P., Shah, N.C., and Wilson, A. (2002) Evolving general practice consultation in Britain: issues of length and context. *BMJ*: 324: 880–882.

Freidin, R.B., Goldman, L., and Cecil, R.R. (1980) Patient-physician concordance in problem identification in the primary care setting. *Ann Intern Med*: 93(3): 490–3

Frenkel, D.N., & Liebman, C.B. (2004) Words that heal. *Annals of Internal Medicine*: 140: 482–483.

Freud, S. (1910) *Two short accounts of psychoanalysis*. London, Hogarth Press, 1997.

Gallagher, T.H., Garbutt, J.M., Waterman, A.D., Flum, D.R., Larson, E.B., Waterman, B.M., Dunagan, W.C., Fraser, V.J., and Levinson, W. (2006) Choosing your words carefully: How physicians would disclose harmful medical errors to patients. *Arch Intern Med*: 166: 1585–1593.

Garg, A., Buckman, R., and Kason, Y. (1997) Teaching medical students how to break bad news. *CMAJ*: 156: 115964.

General Medical Council (2002) *English Language Requirements*. http://www.gmc-uk.org/doctors/registration_applications/language_ proficiency.asp Accessed 1st December 2009.

References

General Medical Council. (2003) *Tomorrow's Doctors* http://www.gmc-uk. org/education/undergraduate/tomorrows_doctors_2003.asp Accessed 23rd November 2009.

General Medical Council. (2006) *Good Medical Practice*. http://www.gmc-uk.org/guidance/good_medical_practice.asp, Accessed 23rd November 2009.

General Medical Council. (2007) *The New Doctor*. http://www.gmc-uk. org/education/postgraduate/new_doctor.asp Accessed 23rd November 2009.

General Medical Council. (2007) *Operationalising Good Medical Practice*. http://www.gmc-uk.org/guidance/good_medical_practice/ operationalising_gmp.asp Accessed 23rd November 2009.

General Medical Council (2009) *Tomorrow's Doctors*. http://www.gmc-uk. org/education/undergraduate/tomorrows_doctors_2009.asp Accessed 30th November 2009.

Gilbert, T. (2009) Introducing compassion focused therapy. *Advances in Psychiatric Treatment*: 15(3): 199–209.

Girgis, A., & Sanson-Fisher, R.W. (1995) Breaking bad news? Consensus guidelines for medical practitioners. *J Clin Oncol*: 13: 2449–2456.

Glaser, V. (2000) Topics in geriatrics: effective approaches to depression in older patients. *Patient Care*: 34(17): 65–70.

Godolphin, W. (2003) The role of risk communication in shared decision making. *BMJ*: 327: 692–693.

Goldacre, M.J., Davidson, J.M., and Lambert, T.W. (2003) Doctors' views of their first year of medical work and postgraduate training in the UK: questionnaire surveys. *BMJ*: 327: 596–7.

Goleman, D. (1998). What makes a leader? *Harvard Business Review*: November–December, 92–102.

Goodyear-Smith, F., & Buetow, S. (2001) Power issues in the doctor-patient relationship. *Health Care Analysis*: 9: 449–462.

Gordon, G.H., Loos, S.K., and Byrne, J. (2000) Physician expressions of uncertainty during patient encounters. *Patient Educ Couns*: 40: 59–65. In print

Graugaard, P.K., & Arnstein, F. (2000) Trait Anxiety and Reactions to Patient-Centered and Doctor-Centered Styles of Communication: An Experimental Study. *Psychosomatic Medicine*: 62: 33–39

Gray, B., & Stoddard, J.J. (1997) Patient-physician pairing: Does racial and ethnic congruity influence selection of a regular physician? *Journal of Community Health*: 22: 247–259.

Greeson, J.M. (2009) Mindfulness research update: 2008. *Complementary Health Practice Review*: 14: 10–18.

Griffin, S.J., Kinmonth, A.L., Veltman, M.W.M., Gillard, S., Grant, J., and Stewart, M. (2004) Effect on health-related outcomes of interventions to alter the interaction between patients and practitioners: a systematic review of trials. *Ann Fam Med*: 2: 595–608.

Griffiths, C.H., Wilson, J.F., Langer, S., and Haist, S.A. (2003) House staff nonverbal communication skills and standardized patient satisfaction. *J Gen Intern Med*.: 18(3): 170–174.

Groene, O., Lombarts, M.J.M.H., Klazinga, N., Alonso, J., Thompson, A., and Suñol, R. (2009) Is patient-centredness in European hospitals related to existing quality improvement strategies? Analysis of a cross-sectional survey (MARQuLS study). *Qual Saf Health Care*: 18: i44–i50.

Groopman, J. (2008) *How Doctors Think*. New York, Mariner Books.

Guerra, C.E., McDonald, V.J., Ravenell, K.L., Asch, D.A., and Shea, J.A. (2008) Effect of race on patients expectations regarding their primary care physicians. *Family Practice*: 25: 49–55.

Gull, S.E. (2002) Communication skills: recognising the difficulties. *The Obstetrician and Gynaecologist*: 4: 107–110.

Haidet, P., & Paterniti, D.A. (2003) "Building" a history rather than "taking" one: A perspective on information sharing during the medical interview. *Archives of Internal Medicine*: 163: 1134–1140.

Haidet, P., Dains, J.E., Paterniti, D.A., Hechtel, L., Chang, T., Tseng, E., and Rogers, J.C. (2002) Medical student attitudes toward the doctor-patient relationship. *Medical Education*: 36: 568–574.

References

Hall, J.A., Roter, D.L., and Rand, C.S. (1981) Communication of affect between patient and physician. *Journal of Health and Social Behavior*: 22: 18–30.

Hall, J.A., Roter, D.L., and Katz, N.R. (1988) Meta-analysis of correlates of provider behaviour in medical encounter. *Med Care*: 26: 657–675.

Hall, J.A., Harrigan, J.A., and Rosenthal, R. (1995) Nonverbal behavior in clinician-patient interaction. *Applied & Preventive Psychology*: 4: 21–37.

Hall, J.A., & Roter, D.L. (2002) Do patients talk differently to male and female physicians? A meta–analytic review. *Patient Education and Counselling*: 48: 217–224.

Hamilton, J., Campos, R., and Creed, F. (1996) Anxiety, depression and management of medically unexplained symptoms in medical clinics. *Journal of the Royal College of Physicians of London*: 30: 18–20

Hampton, J.R., Harrison, M.J.G., Mitchell, J.R., Prichard, J.S., and Seymour, C. (1975) Relative contributions of history taking, physical examination and laboratory investigation to diagnosis and management of medical outpatients. *BMJ*: 2: 486–489.

Hargie, O., Dickson, D., Boohan, M., and Hughes, K. (1998) A survey of communication skills training in UK schools of medicine: present practices and prospective proposals. *Medical Education*: 32: 25–34.

Hargie, O., & Dickson, D. (2004) *Skilled Interpersonal Communication: Research, Theory and Practice*. East Sussex, Routledge.

Harrigan, J.A., Oxman, T.E., and Rosenthal, R. (1985) Rapport expressed through nonverbal behaviour. *Journal of Nonverbal Behavior*: 9: 95–110.

Haskard, K.B., Williams, S.L., DiMatteo, M.R., Rosenthal, R., White, M.K., and Goldstein, M.G. (2008) Physician and Patient Communication Training in Primary Care: Effects on Participation and Satisfaction. *Health Psychology*: 27: 513–522.

Haynes, R.B., McKibbon, K.A., and Kanani, R. (1996) Systematic review of randomised trials of interventions to assist patients to follow prescriptions for medications. *The Lancet*: 348: 383–387.

Healthcare Commission Performance ratings 2005. http://ratings2005.healthcarecommission.org.uk/ Accessed November 2009.

Heath, C. (1984) Participation in the medical consultation: the co-ordination of verbal and non-verbal behaviour between the doctor and the patient. *Sociol Health Illness*: 6: 311–338.

Heath, I. (2003) A wolf in sheep's clothing: a critical look at the ethics of drug taking. *BMJ*: 327: 856–858.

Helft, P.R., Hlubocky, F., and Daugherty, C.K. (2003) American oncologists´ views of internet use by cancer patients: A mail survey of American society of clinical oncology members. *J Clin Oncol*: 21: 942–947.

Hickson, G.B., Federspiel, C.F., Pichert, J.W., Miller, C.S., Gauld-Jaeger, J., and Bost, P. (2002) Patient complaints and malpractice risk. *JAMA*: 287(22): 3003.

Holman, D.H. (2000) A dialogical approach to skill and skilled activity. *Human Relations*: 53(7): 957–980.

Holman, H., & Lorig, K. (2000) Patients as partners in managing chronic disease. *BMJ*: 320: 526–527.

Holmes-Rovner, M., Valade, D., Orlowski, C., Draus, C., Nabozny-Valerio, B., and Keiser, S. (2000) Implementing shared decision making in routine practice: barriers and opportunities. *Health Expect*: 3: 182–191.

Hulsman, R.L., Ros, W.J., Winnubst, J.A., and Bensing, J.M. (1999) Teaching clinically experienced physicians communication skills. A review of evaluation studies. *Med Educ*: 33: 655–668.

Hulsman, R.L., Ros, W.J., Winnubst, J.A., and Bensing, J.M. (2002) The effectiveness of a computer-assisted instruction programme on communication skills of medical specialists in oncology. *Med Educ*: 36(2): 125–134.

Hurwitz, B., & Vass, A. (2002) What's a good doctor, and how can you make one? *BMJ*: 325: 667–668.

Idler, E.L., & Kasl, S. (1991) Health perceptions and survival: Do global evaluations of health status really predict mortality? *Journal of Gerontology*: 46: S55–65.

Ihler, E. (2003) Patient-physician communication. *JAMA*: 289: 92.

References

Institute of Medicine (2001) *Crossing the quality chasm: A new health system for the 21st century*. Washington DC, National Academy Press.

Irwin, R.S., & Richardson, N.D. (2006) Patient-focused care. *Chest*: 130: 73S–82S.

Jackson, J.L., Chamberlin, J., and Kroenke, K. (2001) Predictors of patient satisfaction. *Soc Sci Med*: 609–620

Jenkins, V., & Fallowfield, L. (2002) Can communication skills training alter physicians beliefs and behaviour in clinics. *Journal of Clinical Oncology*: 20(3): 765–769.

Jones, J. (2003) Prescribing and taking medicines. *BMJ*: 327: 819–820.

Joos, S.K., Hickam, D.H., and Borders, L.M. (1993) Patients' desires and satisfaction in general medicine clinics. *Public Health Rep*: 108: 751–759.

Joos, S.K., Hickam, D.H., Gordon, G.H., and Baker, L.H. (1996) Effects of a physician communication intervention on patient care outcomes. *J. Gen. Int. Med.*: 11: 147–155.

Jung, H.P., Wensing, M., and Grol, R. (1997) What makes a good general practitioner: do patients and doctors have different views? *Br J Gen Pract*: 47(425): 805–9.

Kalet, A., Pugnaire, M.P., Cole-Kelly, K., Janicik, R., Ferrara, E., Lipkin, M., and Lazare, A. (2004) Teaching communication in clinical clerkships: models from the Macy initiative in health communication. *Academic Medicine*: 76: 511–520.

Kaplan, S.H., Greenfield, S., and Ware, J.E Jr. (1989) Impact of the doctor-patient relationship on the outcomes of chronic disease. In: Stewart, M., & Roter, D. editors, *Communicating with Medical Patients*, Beverley Hills, CA, Sage Publications, pp 228–245.

Kaplan, S.H., Greenfield, S., and Ware, J.E. Jr. (1989a) Assessing the effects of physician-patient interactions on the outcomes of chronic disease. *Med Care*: 27(7): 679.

Kaplan, S.K., Greenfield, S., Gandek, B., Rogers, W.H., Ware, J.E. (1996) Characteristics of physicians with participatory decision-making styles. *Ann Intern Med*: 124: 497–504.

Kaptchuk, T.J. (2002) The placebo effect in alternative medicine: Can the performance of a healing ritual have clinical significance? *Ann Intern Med*: 136: 817–825.

Karel, M. J. (2007) Culture and medical decision making in *Changes in decision-making capacity in older adults: Assessment and intervention* p145–147: United Kingdom, Wiley.

Keller, V.F., & Carroll, J.G. (1994) A new model for physician-patient communication. *Patient Educ Couns*: 23: 131–140.

Kennedy, J. (2002). Physicians' feelings about themselves and their patients. *JAMA*: 287: 1113.

Kennedy, J.G. (2003) "Doc, tell me what I need to know" – a doctor's perspective. *BMJ*: 327: 862–863.

Kessels, R.P. (2003) Patients' memory for medical information. *Journal of the Royal Society of Medicine*: 96(5): 219–22.

Kidd, J., Patel, V., Peile, E., and Carter, Y. (2005) Clinical and communication skills. *BMJ*: 330: 374–375.

Kindelan, K., & Kent, G. (1987) Concordance between patients' information preferences and general practitioners' perceptions. *Psychol Health*: 1: 399–409.

Kinmonth, A.L., Woodcock, A., Griffin, S., Spiegal, N., and Campbell, M.J. (1998) Randomised controlled trial of patient-centred care of diabetes in general practice: impact on current wellbeing and future disease risk. *BMJ*: 317: 1202–1208.

Kinnersley, P., Stott, N., Peters, T.J., and Harvey, I. (1999) The patient-centredness of consultations and outcome in primary care. *Br J Gen Pract*: 49(446): 711–716.

Kinnersely, P., Edwards, A., Hood, K., Ryan, R., Prout, H., Cadbury, N., MacBeth, F., Butow, P., and Butler, C. (2008) Interventions before consultations to help patients address their information needs by encouraging question asking: systematic review. *BMJ*: 337: a485.

Kinnersely, P., & Edwards, A. (2008) Complaints against doctors. *BMJ*: 336: 841–2

References

Kinnersley, P., & Spencer, J. (2008) Communication skills teaching comes of age. *Medical Education*: 42: 1053–1053.

Kirsner, J.B. (2009) The most powerful therapeutic force. *JAMA*: 287(15): 1909–1910.

Kivits, J. (2006) Informed patients and the internet. *Journal of Health Psychology*: 11(2): 269–282.

Klyman, C.M., Browne, M., Austad, C., Spindler, E.J., and Spindler, A.C. (2008) A Workshop Model for Educating Medical Practitioners about Optimal Treatment of Difficult-to-Manage Patients: Utilization of Transference-Countertransference. *Journal of the American Academy of Psychoanalysis and Dynamic Psychiatry*: 36: 61–77.

Korsch, B.M., Gozzi, E.K., and Francis, V. (1968) Gaps in doctor- patient communication. *Pediatrics*: 42: 855–871.

Korsch, B.M. (1989) The past and the future of research in doctor-patient relations. In: Stewart, M., & Roter, D. editors, *Communicating with Medical Patients*: Beverley Hills, CA, Sage Publications, 1989 pp 246–251.

Kravitz, R.L., Hays, R.D., Sherbourne, C.D., DiMatteo, M.R., Rogers, W.H., Ordway, L., and Greenfield, S. (1993) Recall of recommendations and adherence to advice among patients with chronic medical conditions. *Arch Intern Med*: 153(16): 1869–1878.

Kravitz, R..L, Cope, D.W., Bhrany, V., and Leake, B. (1994) Internal medicine patients' expectations for care during office visits. J *Gen Intern Med*: 9: 75–81.

Kroenke, K. (2001) Studying symptoms: sampling and measurement issues. *Ann Intern Med*: 134: 844–55.

Kroenke, K., & Harris, L. (2001) Symptoms research: A fertile field. *Ann Intern Med*: 134: 851–853.

Kurtz, S., Silverman, J., and Draper, J. (2005) *Teaching and Learning Communication Skills in Medicine (Second Edition)*. Oxford, Radcliffe Publishing.

Landy, F.J. (2005) Some historical and scientific issues related to research on emotional intelligence. *Journal of Organizational Behavior*: 26: 411–424.

Lang, F., Floyd, M.R., Beine, K.L., and Buck, P. (2002) Sequenced questioning to elicit patients´ perspective on illness: effects on information disclosure, patient satisfaction and time expenditure. *Family Medicine*: 34: 325–330.

Langiewitz, W.A., Eich, P., Kiss, A., and Wössmer, B. (1998) Improving communication skills – A randomized controlled behaviourally oriented intervention study for residents in internal medicine. *Psychosomatic Medicine*: 60: 258–276.

Langiewitz, W., Denz, M., Keller, A., Kiss, A., Ruttiman, S., and Wössmer, B. (2002) Spontaneous talking time at start of consultation in outpatient clinic: cohort study. *BMJ*: 325: 682–683.

Larsen, K.M., & Smith, C.K. (1981) Assessment of nonverbal communication in the patient-physician interview. *J Fam Pract*: 12: 481–488.

Larson, E.B., & Yao, X. (2005) Clinical empathy as an emotional labor in the patient-physician relationship. *JAMA*: 293(9): 1100–1106.

Launer, J. (2007) *How not to be a doctor*. London, Royal Society of Medicine Press.

Lazare, A., Eisenthal, S., and Wasserman, L. (1975) The customer approach to patienthood: attending to patient requests in a walk-in clinic. *Arch Gen Psychiatry*: 32: 553–8.

Lefer, J. (2006) The Psychoanalyst at the Medical Bedside. *Journal of the American Academy of Psychoanalysis and Dynamic Psychiatry*: 34: 75–81

Lehmann, L.S., Brancati, F.L., Chen, M.C., Roter, D., and Dobs, A.S. (1997) The effect of bedside case presentations on patients perceptions of their medical care. *NEJM*: 336: 1150–1156.

Levenstein, J.H., Brown, J.B., Weston, W.W., Stewart, M., McCracken, E.C., and McWhinney, I. (1989) Patient-Centred clinical interviewing. In: Stewart, M., & Roter, D. editors, *Communicating with Medical Patients*, Beverley Hills, CA, Sage Publications, pp 107–120

Levinson, W., Stiles, W.B., Inui, T.S., and Engle, R. (1993) Physician frustration in communicating with patients. *Med Care*: 31: 285–295.

Levinson, W., Roter, D.L., Mullooly, J.P., Dull, V.T., and Frankel, M. (1997) Physician-patient communication. The relationship with malpractice claims among primary care physicians and surgeons. *JAMA*: 277(7): 553–559.

References

Levinson, W., Gorawara-Bhat, R., and Lamb. (2000) J. A study of patient clues and physician responses in primary care and surgical settings. *JAMA*: 284: 1021–1027.

Levinson, W., Cohen, M.S., Brady, D., and Duffy, F.D. (2001) To change or not to change: "Sounds like you have a dilemma". *Annals of Internal Medicine*: 135(5): 386–391.

Levinson, W., & Lurie, N. (2004) When most doctors are women: What lies ahead? *Ann Intern Med*: 141: 471–474.

Levinson, W., Kao, A., Kuby, A., and Thisted, R.A. (2005) Not all patients want to participate in decision making: a national study of public preferences. *JGIM*: 20: 531–535.

Lewin, S., Skea, Z., Entwistle, V.A., Zwarenstein, M., and Dick, J. (2001) Interventions for providers to promote a patient-centred approach in clinical consultations. *Cochrane Database of Systematic Reviews 2001*, Issue 4. Art No: CD003267. DOI: 10.1002/14651858.CD003267.

Lewis, D.K, Robinson, J., and Wilkinson, E. (2003) Factors involved in deciding to start preventive treatment: qualitative study of clinicians' and lay people's attitudes. *BMJ*: 327: 841–5.

Ley, P. (1988) *Communicating with Patients: Improving communication, satisfaction and compliance*. London, Croom Helm.

Ley, P. (1998) The use and improvement of written communication in mental health care and promotion. *Psychology, Health & Medicine*: 3: 19–53.

Leydon, G.M., Boulton, M., Moynihan, C., Jones, A., Mossman, J., Boudioni, M., and McPherson, K. (2000) Cancer patients information needs and information seeking behaviour: in depth interview study. *BMJ*: 320: 909–913.

Lipkin, M.Jr. (1996) Physician-patient interaction in reproductive counselling. *Obstetrics & Gynaecology*: 88(3): 31S–40S.

Little, P., Everitt, H., Williamson, I., Warner, G., Moore, M., Gould, C., Ferrier, K., and Payne, S. (2001a) Preferences of patients for patient-centred approach to consultation in primary care: observational study. *BMJ*: 322: 468.

Little, P., Everitt, H., Williamson, I., Warner, G., Moore, M., Gould, C., Ferrier, K., and Payne, S. (2001b) Observational study of effect of patient-centredness and positive approach on outcomes of general practice consultations. *BMJ*: 323: 908–911.

Littlejohn, S.W., & Foss, K.A. (2005) *Theories of Human Communication. (8th Edition)*: United Kingdom, Thomson Wadsworth.

Locke, E.A. (2005) Why emotional intelligence is an invalid concept. *Journal of Organizational Behavior*: 26: 425–431

Longhurst, M.F. (1989) Physician self-awareness: The neglected insight. In: Stewart, M., & Roter, D. editors, *Communicating with Medical Patients*, Beverley Hills, CA, Sage Publications, pp 64–72

Lowry, J., & Cripps, J. (2005) Results of the online EWTD trainee survey. *Bull R Coll Surgeons Engl*: 87: 86–7.

Macdonald, E. (2004) *Difficult conversations in medicine*. Oxford, Oxford University Press.

MacDonald, R. (2002) This Week. *BMJ Careers*: 7 December: s191

Mager, W.M., & Andrykowski, M.A. (2002) Communication in the cancer 'bad news' consultation: patient perceptions and psychological adjustment. *Psycho-Oncology*: 11(1): 35–46.

Maguire, P., Clarke, D., & Jolly, B. (1977) An experimental comparison of three courses in history-taking skills for medical students. *Medical Education*: 11: 175–182.

Maguire, P. (1985) Barriers to psychological care of the dying. *BMJ*: 291: 1711–3.

Maguire, P., Fairbairn, S., and Fletcher, C. (1986) Consultation skills of young doctors: 1—Benefits of feedback training in interviewing as students persist. *BMJ (Clin Res Ed)*: 292: 1573–1576.

Maguire, P., Fairbairn, S., and Fletcher, C. (1989) Consultation skills of young doctors – Benefits of undergraduate feedback training in interviewing. In: Stewart, M., & Roter, D. editors, *Communicating with Medical Patients*, London, Sage Publications, pp 124–137

References

Maguire, P., Booth, K., Elliott, C., and Jones, B. (1996a) Helping health professionals involved in cancer care acquire key interviewing skills – the impact of workshops. *Eur J Cancer*: 32A: 1486–1489.

Maguire, P., Faulkner, A., Booth, K., Elliott, C., and Hillier, V. (1996b) Helping cancer patients disclose their concern. *Eur J Cancer*: 32A: 78–81.

Maguire, P. (2000) *Communication Skills for Doctors*. London, Arnold.

Maguire, P., & Pitceathly, C. (2002) Key communication skills and how to acquire them. *BMJ*: 325: 697–700.

Makoul, G. (2001) The SEGUE framework for teaching and assessing communication skills. *Patient Educ Couns*: 45: 23–34

Makoul, G., & Curry, R.H. (2007) The value of assessing and addressing communication skills. *JAMA*: 298(9): 1057–1059.

Marinker, M., & Shaw, J. (2003) Not to be taken as directed. *BMJ*: 326: 348–349.

Martin, T.N. & Hafer, J.C. (2009) Models of emotional intelligence, spiritual intelligence and performance: a test of Tischler, Biberman, and McKeage. *Journal of Management, Spirituality & Religion*: 6: 247–257

Marvel, M.K., Epstein, R.M., Flowers, K., and Beckman, H.B. (1999) Soliciting the patients agenda. *JAMA*: 281: 283–287.

Mast, M.S., Hall, J.A., Kockner, C., and Choi, E. (2008) Physician gender affects how physician nonverbal behaviour is related to patient satisfaction. *Medical Care*: 46(12): 1212–1218.

Matthews, D.A., Suchman, A.L., and Branch, W.T. Jr. (1993) Making "connexions": Enhancing the therapeutic potential of patient-clinician relationships. *Annals of Internal Medicine*: 118: 973–977.

Maynard, D.W. & Heritage, J. (2005) Conversation analysis, doctor–patient interaction and medical communication. *Medical Education*: 39: 428–435

Mayou, R., Williamson, B., and Foster, A. (1976) Attitudes and advice after myocardial infarction. *BMJ*: 1: 1577–1579.

McKinstry, B. (2000) Do patients wish to be involved in decision making in the consultation? A cross sectional survey with video vignettes. *BMJ*: 321: 867–871.

McManus, I.C., Winder, B.C., and Gordon, D. (2002) The causal links between stress and burnout in a longitudinal study of UK doctors. *The Lancet*: 359: 2089–2090.

McMullen, B. (2002) Cognitive Intelligence. *BMJ*: 325: S193–4.

McWhinney, I. (1989) The need for a transformed clinical method. In: Stewart, M., & Roter, D. editors, *Communicating with Medical Patients*. Beverley Hills, CA, Sage Publications, pp 25–40.

Mehrabian, A. (1972) *Nonverbal communication*. Chicago, Aldine-Atherton.

Melchiode, G.A. (1979) Psychoanalytic teaching in medical education. *The American Journal of Psychiatry*: 136(8): 1071–1073.

Mercer, S.W., Watt, G.C.M., and Reilly, D. (2001) Empathy is important for enablement. *BMJ*: 332: 865.

Mercer, S.W., & Howie, J.G.R. (2006) CQI–2 – a new measure of holistic interpersonal care in primary care consultations. *Br J Gen Pract*: 56: 262–268.

Meryn, S. (1998) Improving doctor patient communication. *BMJ*: 316: 1922.

Mizco, N., Segrin, C., and Allspach, L.E. (2001) Relationship between nonverbal sensitivity, encoding, and relational satisfaction. *Communication Reports*: 14(1): 39.

Mollon, P. (2001) The current role of psychoanalysis and psychotherapy in primary care. *Primary Care Psychiatry*: 7(2): 43–47.

Murray, A., Pounder, R., Mather, H., and Black, Dame C. (2005) Junior doctor' shifts and sleep deprivation: The European working time directive may put doctors' and patients' lives at risk. *BMJ*: 330: 1404.

Neighbour, R. (2005) *The Inner Consultation: how to develop an effective and intuitive consulting style*. UK: Radcliffe Publishing Ltd.

Newell, S., Sanson-Fisher, R.W., and Bonaventura, A. (1998) How well do medical oncologists' perceptions reflect their patients' reported physical and psycho-social problems? Data from a survey of five oncologists. *Cancer*: 83: 1640.

References

NHS Institute for Innovation and Improvement and the Academy of Medical Royal Colleges. (2008) Medical Leadership Competency Framework. http://www.institute.nhs.uk/assessment_tool/general/medical_leadership_competency_framework_-_homepage.html Accessed 23rd November 2009.

National Institute for Clinical Excellence (NICE). (2005) *Violence: the short-term management of disturbed/violent behaviour in psychiatric in-patient settings and emergency departments.* http://www.guideline.gov/summary/summary.aspx?doc_id=6570&nbr=4132&ss=15 Accessed 2nd December 2009.

National Institute for Clinical Excellence (NICE) *clinical guideline 76 (2009) Medicines adherence.* London: National Institute for Health and Clinical Excellence.

Nimnuan, C., Hotopf, M., and Wessely, S. (2000) Medically unexplained symptoms: how often and why are they missed? *Q J Med*: 93: 21–28.

Novack, D.H., Volk, G., Drossman, D.A., and Lipkin, M. (1993) Medical interviewing and interpersonal skills teaching in US medical schools: practice, problems and promise. *JAMA*: 269: 2101–5.

Novack, D.H., Suchman, A.L., Clark, W., Epstein, R.M., Najberg, E., and Kaplan, C. (1997) Calibrating the physician. Personal awareness and effective patient care. Working group on promoting physician personal awareness, American academy on physician and patient. *JAMA*: 278: 502–509.

O'Dowd, T.C. (1988) Five years of heartsink patients in general practice. *BMJ*: 297:528–30.

O'Connor, A.M., Rostom, A., Fiset, V., Tetroe, J., Entwistle, V., Llewellyn-Thomas, H., Holmes-Rovner, M., Barry, M., and Jones, J. (1999) Decision aids for patients facing health treatment or screening decisions: systematic review. *BMJ*: 319: 731–4.

Ohtaki, S., Ohtaki, T., and Fetters, M.D. (2003) Doctor-patient communication: a comparison of the USA and Japan. *Family Practice*: 20: 276–282.

Orlander, J.D., Fincke, B.G., Hermanns, D., and Johnson, G.A. (2002) Medical residents'first clearly remembered experiences of giving bad news. *J Gen Intern Med*: 17: 825–831.

Ospina, M.B., Bond, K., Karkhaneh, M., Tjosvold, L., Vandermeer, B., Liang, Y., Bialy, L., Hooton, N., Buscemi, N., Dryden, D.M., and Klassen, T.P. (2007) Meditation practices for health: state of the research. *Evidence Report/Technology Assessment*: 155: 1–263

Pace, T.W.W., Negi, L.T., Adame, D.D., Cole, S.P., Sivilli, T.I., Brown, T.D., Issa, M.J., and Raison, C.L. (2009) Effect of compassion meditation on neuroendocrine, innate immune and behavioral responses to psychosocial stress. *Psychoneuroendocrinology*: 34: 87–98.

Pena Dolhun, E., Munoz, C., Grumbach, K. (2003) Cross-cultural education in U.S. Medical schools: Development of an assessment tool. *Academic Medicine*: 78: 615–622.

Pendleton, D., Schofield, T., Tate, P., and Havelock, P. (2003) *The New Consultation*. Oxford, Oxford University Press.

Pennebaker, J., & Francis, M. (1996) Cognitive, emotional and language processes in disclosure. *Cognition & Emotion*: 10(6): 601–626.

Perez, J.C. (2004) Healing presence. *Care Management Journals*: 5: 41–46.

Perrin, S. (1997) Managing violence and aggression on a renal unit. *EDTNA-ERCA Journal*: 23: 34–36.

Peterson, M.C., Holbrook, J., Von Hales, D., Smith, N.L., and Staker, L,V. (1992) Contributions of the history, physical examination and laboratory investigation in making medical diagnoses. *West J Med*: 156: 163–5.

Pinock, S. (2004) Poor communication lies at the heart of NHS complaints, says ombudsman. *BMJ*: 328: 10.

Placek, J.T., & Eberhart, T.L. (1996) Breaking bad news: A review of the literature. *JAMA*: 276: 496–502.

Platt, F.W., & McMath, J.C. (1979) Clinical hypocompetence: the interview. *Annals of Internal Medicine*: 91: 898–902.

Platt, F.W., Gaspar, D.L., Coulehan, J.L., Fox, L., Adler, A.J., Weston, W.W., Smith, R.C., and Stewart, M. (2001) "Tell me about yourself": The patient–centred interview. *Annals of Internal Medicine*: 134: 1079–1085.

Poole, A.D., & Sanson-Fisher, R.W. (1979) Understanding the patient: A neglected aspect of medical education. *Social Science*: 13A: 37–43.

Praissman, S. (2008) Mindfulness-based stress reduction: A literature review and clinician's guide. *Journal of the American Academy of Nurse Practitioners*: 20: 212–216.

Preven, D.W., Kachur, E.K., Kupfer, R.B., and Waters, J.A. (1986) Interviewing skills of first-year medical students. *Journal of Medical Education*: 61(10): 842–4

Prior, A. (1993) Personal view: More than a physical disease. *BMJ*: 304:61.

Rafferty, A.M., Ball, J., and Aiken, L.H. (2001) Are teamwork and professional autonomy compatible, and do they result in improved hospital care? *Quality in Health Care*: 10: Suppl. 2(ii32–ii37)

Ramirez, A.J., Graham, J., Richards, M.A., Cull, A., and Gregory, W.M. (1996) Mental health of hospital consultants: the effects of stress and satisfaction at work. *The Lancet*: 347: 724–728.

Reid, S., Wessely, S., and Crayford, T. (2001) Medically unexplained symptoms in frequent attendees of secondary health care: retrospective cohort study. *BMJ*: 322: 767–769.

Rees, C., & Sheard, C. (2002) The relationship between medical students attitudes towards communication skills learning and their demographic and education-related characteristics. *Medical Education*: 36: 1017–1027.

Reid, S., Wessely, S., Crayford, T., and Hotopf, M. (2001) Medically unexplained symptoms in frequent attenders of secondary health care. *BMJ*: 322: 767–769.

Rew, M., & Ferns, T. (2005) A balanced approach to dealing with violence and aggression at work. *British Journal of Nursing*: 14: 227–32.

Reynolds, W.J., & Scott, B. (2000) Do nurses and other professional helpers normally display much empathy? *Journal of Advanced Nursing*: 31(1): 226–234.

Rice, B. (2001) What doctors want most from practice. *Medical Economics*: 78: 38.

Richards, T. (1990) Chasms in communication – still occur too often. *BMJ*: 301: 1407–8.

Richter, D. (2006) Non-physical conflict management and de-escalation. In Richter, D., & Whittington, R. *Violence in mental health settings: Causes, consequences, management*. New York, Springer-Verlag, pp125–141.

Ridsdale, L., Morgan, M., and Morris, R. (1992) Doctors interviewing technique and its response to different booking time. *Family Practice*: 9: 57–60.

Roberts, C., Cox, C., Reintgen, D., Baile, W., and Gilbertini, M. (1994) Influence of physicians communication on newly diagnosed breast patients' psychologic adjustment and decision-making. *Cancer*: 74: 336–341.

Rocca, P., Villari, V., and Bogetto, F. (2006) Managing the aggressive and violent patient in the psychiatric emergency. *Progress in Neuro-Psychopharmacology & Biological Psychiatry*: 30: 586–98.

Rogers, M.S., & Todd, C.J. (2000) The ´right kind´of pain: talking about symptoms in outpatient oncology consultations. *Palliative Medicine*: 14: 299–307.

Rollnick, S., & Miller, W.R. (1995). What is motivational interviewing? *Behavioural and Cognitive Psychotherapy*: 23: 325–334.

Rollnick, S., Butler, C.C., McCambridge, J., Kinnersley, P., Elwyn, G., and Resnicow, K. (2005) Consultations about changing behaviour. *BMJ*: 331: 961–963.

Rosen, R., & Dewar, S. (2004) *On being a doctor: redefining medical professionalism for better patient care*. London, King's Fund.

Roter, D.L., & Hall, J.A. (1987) Physicians interviewing styles and medical information obtained from patients. *J Gen Intern Med*: 2: 329–329.

Roter, D. (1989) Which facets of communication have strong effects on outcome – A meta-analysis. In: Stewart, M., & Roter, D. editors, *Communicating with Medical Patients*, Beverley Hills, CA, Sage Publications, pp 183–196.

Roter, D.L., Hall, J.A., Kern, D.E., Barker, L.R., Cole, K.A. and Roca, R.P. (1995) Improving physicians interviewing skills and reducing patients' emotional distress. A randomized clinical trial. *Arch Intern Med*: 155(17): 1877–1884.

Roter, D. (2000) The enduring and evolving nature of the patient-physician relationship. *Patient Educ Couns*: 39: 5–15.

References

Roter, D.L., Hall, J.A., and Aoki, Y. (2002) Physician gender effects in medical communication: A meta-analytic review. *JAMA*: 288(6): 756–764.

Roter, D.L., & Hall, J.A. (2006) *Doctors Talking with Patients/Patients Talking with Doctors*. London, Praeger.

Roter, D.L., Geller, G., Bernhardt, B.A., Larson, S.M., and Doksum, T. (1999) Effect of obstetrician gender on communication and patient satisfaction. *Obstetrics & Gynaecology*: 93: 635–641.

Royal College of Physicians (1997) *Improving communication between doctors and patients*. London, Royal College of Physicians.

Royal College of Physicians (2005) *Doctors in Society. Medical professionalism in a changing world. Report of a working party*. London, Royal College of Physicians.

Royal College of Surgeons of England. (2005) *Surgical Training Seriously Compromised by European Working Time Directive*. 24th February 2005. http://www.rcseng.ac.uk/media/medianews/Surgicaltrainingcompromisedbyworkingtimedirective Accessed 23rd November 2009.

Royal College of Physicians. (2006) *Census of Consultant Physicians in the UK, 2005*. London, Royal College of Physicians.

Ruusuvuori, J. (2001) Looking means listening: coordinating displays of engagement in doctor-patient interaction. *Soc Sci Med*: 52: 1093–1108.

Salinsky, J., & Sackin, P. (2000) *What are you feeling, Doctor*? Oxford, Radcliffe Medical Press.

Salmon, P., Sephton, S., Weissbecker, I., Hoover, K., Ulmer, C., and Studts, J.L. (2004) Mindfulness meditation in clinical practice. *Cognitive and Behavioral Practice*: 11: 434–446.

Salmon, P., & May, C.R. (1995) Patients' influence on doctors' behaviour: a case study of patient strategies in somatisation. *International Journal of Psychiatry and Medicine*: 25: 319–329.

Salovey, P., & Mayer, J.D. (1990). Emotional intelligence. *Imagination, Cognition, and Personality*: 9: 185–211.

Sanchez, M.M. (2001) Effects of assertive communication between doctors and patients in public health outpatient surgeries in the city of Seville (Spain). *Social Behavior and Personality*: 29: 63–70.

Sanchez-Menegay, C., & Stalder, H. (1994) Do physicians take into account Patients' expectations? *J Gen Intern Med*: 9: 404–406.

Sanson-Fisher, R.W., & Poole, A.D. (1978) Training medical students to empathize. An experimental study. *Medical Journal of Australia*: 1: 473–476.

Sardell, A.N., & Trierweiler, S.J. (1993) Disclosing the cancer diagnosis: Procedures that influence patient hopefulness. *Cancer*: 72: 3355–3365.

Saunders, C. (1996) Into the Valley of the Shadow of Death: A personal therapeutic journey. *BMJ*: 313: 1599–1601.

Savage, R., & Armstrong, D. (1990) Effect of a general practitioner's consulting style on patients' satisfaction: a controlled study. *BMJ*: 310: 968–970.

Schmid, M., Hall, J.A., and Roter, D.L. (2007) Disentangling physician sex and physician communication style: their effects on patient satisfaction in a virtual medical visit. *Patient Education & Counseling*: 68(1): 16–22.

Schofield, T., Elwyn, G., Edwards, A., and Visser, A. (2003) Shared decision making. *Patient Educ Couns*: 50: 229–230.

Schouten, B.C., & Meeuwesen, L. (2006) Cultural differences in medical communication: A review of the literature. *Patient Education and Counseling*: 64: 21–34.

Schreiner, I., & Malcolm, J.P. (2008) The benefits of mindfulness meditation: Changes in emotional states of depression, anxiety, and stress. *Behaviour Change*: 25: 156–168.

Schutz, A. (1998) Assertive, offensive, protective and defensive styles of self-presentation: A taxonomy. *The Journal of Psychology*: 132: 611–628.

Secretary of State for Health. (2000) *The NHS Plan*. London, Stationery Office.

Sedgwick, P., & Hall, A. (2003) Teaching medical students and doctors how to communicate risk. *BMJ*: 327: 694–695.

References

Shah, R., & Ogden. J. (2006) 'What's in a face?' the role of doctor ethnicity, age and gender in the formation of patients' judgements: An experimental study. *Patient Education and Counseling*: 60: 136–141.

Shapiro, S.L., Oman, D., Thoresen, C.E., Plante, T.G., and Flinders, T. (2008) Cultivating mindfulness: effects on well-being. *Journal of Clinical Psychology*: 64: 840–62.

Shilling, V., Jenkins, V., and Fallowfield, L. (2003) Factors affecting patient and clinician satisfaction with the clinical consultation: can communication skills training for clinicians improve satisfaction? *Psycho-Oncology*: 12: 699–611.

Shooter, M. (2002) Students heads are so full of lists they have forgotten how to listen. *BMJ*: 325: 677.

Silverman, J., Kurtz, S. & Draper, J. (2005) *Skills for Communicating with Patients Second Edition*. Oxford, Radcliffe Publishing.

Simpson, M., Buckman, R., Stewart, M., Maguire, P., Lipkin, M., Novack, D., and Till, J. (1991) Doctor-patient communication: the Toronto consensus. *BMJ*: 303: 1385–1387.

Simpson, J.G., Furnace, J., Crosby, J., Cumming, A.D., Evans, P.A., Friedman, M., David, B., Harden, R.M., Lloyd, D., McKenzie, H., McLachlan, J.C., McPhate, G.F., Percy-Robb, I.W., and MacPherson, S.G. (2002) The Scottish doctor/learning outcomes for the medical undergraduate in Scotland: a foundation for competent and reflective practitioners. *Medical Teacher*: 24: 136–143.

Serour, M., Al Othman, H., and Al Khalifah, G. (2009) Difficult patients or difficult doctors: An analysis of problematic consultations. *European Journal of General Medicine*: 6(2): 34–40.

Skelton, J.R., & Hobbs, F.D.R. (1999) Concordancing. Use of language-based research in medical communication. *The Lancet*: 353: 108–111.

Skelton, J.R., Wearn, A.M., Hobbs, R. (2002) 'I' and 'we': a concordancing analysis of how doctors and patients use first person pronouns in primary care consultations. *Family Practice*: 19: 484–488.

Sloane, J.A. (1993) Offenses and defenses against patients: a psychoanalyst's view of the borderline between empathic failure and malpractice. *Can J Psychiatry*: 38: 265–273.

Smith, R.C. (1984) Teaching interviewing skills to medical students: the issue of 'countertransference'. *Journal of Medical Education*: 59(7): 582–8.

Smith, R.C. (1986) Unrecognized responses and feelings of residents and fellows during interviews of patients. *Journal of Medical Education*: 61(12): 982–4.

Smith, R.C., & Hoppe, R.B. (1991) The patient's story: integrating the patient and physician centred approaches to interviewing. *Ann Intern Med*: 115: 471–477.

Smith, S. (1995) Dealing with the difficult patient. *Postgraduate Medical Journal*: 71: 653–657.

Smith, R. (2003) An extreme failure of concordance. *BMJ*: 327: 0.

Smith, S., Mitchell, C., and Bowler, S. (2008) Standard versus patient-centred asthma education in the emergency department: a randomised study. *Eur Respir J*: 31: 990–997.

Spiro, H. (1992) What is empathy and can it be taught? *Ann. Intern. Med.*: 16: 843–846.

Spitzberg, B.H. (1983) Communication competence as knowledge, skill and impression. *Communication Education*: 32: 323–329.

Squier, R. (1990) A model of empathic understanding and adherence to treatment regimes in practitioner-patient relationships. *Social Science Medicine*: 30: 325–339.

Starfield, B., Wray, C., Hess, K., Gross, R., Birk, P.S., and D'Lugoff, B.C. (1981) The influence of patient-practitioner agreement on outcome of care. *Am J Public Health*: 71: 127–132.

Stevens, J. (1974) Brief Encounter. *Journal of Royal College of General Practice*: 24: 5–22.

Stewart, M.A., McWhinney, I.R., and Buck, C.W. (1979) The doctor/patient relationship and its effect upon outcome. *J Royal Coll Gen Pract*: 29: 77–82.

Stewart, M.A. (1985) *Comparison of two methods of analysing doctor-patient communication*. Paper presented at the North American Primary Care Research Group Conference, Seattle, 14–17 April 1985.

References

Stewart, M., & Roter, D. (1989) *Communicating with Medical Patients*. Sage Publications, London.

Stewart, M.A. (1995) Effective physician–patient communication and health outcomes: a review. *Canadian Medical Association Journal*: 152: 1423–1433.

Stewart, M., Brown, J.B., Boon, H., Galajda, J., Meredith, L., and Sangster, M. (1999) Evidence on patient-doctor communication. *Cancer Prev Control*: 3: 25–30.

Stewart, M., Brown, J.B., Donner, A., McWhinney, I.R., Oates, J., Weston, W.W., and Jordan, J. (2000) The impact of patient-centred care on outcomes. *J Fam Pract*: 49: 796–804.

Stewart, M. (2001) Towards a global definition of patient-centred care. *BMJ*: 322: 444–445.

Stewart, M. (2004) Continuity, Care and Commitment: The course of the patient-clinician relationships. *Annals of Family Medicine*: 2: 388–390.

Stewart, M. (2005) Reflections on the doctor-patient relationship: for evidence and experience. *Br J Gen Pract*: 55: 793–801.

Strous, R.D., Ulman, A-M., and Kotler, M. (2006) The hateful patient revisited: Relevance for 21st century medicine: *European Journal of Internal Medicine*: 17(6): 387–393.

Suchman, A.L. (2003) Research on patient-clinician relationships: celebrating success and identifying the next scope of work. *Gen Intern Med*: 18(8): 677–678.

Sullivan, P., & Buske, L. (1998) Results from CMA´s huge 1998 physician survey point to a dispirited profession. *CMAJ*: 159: 525–528.

Svarstad, B.L. (1974) *The Doctor-Patient Encounter: an observational study of communication and outcome*. Madison, WI, University of Wisconsin.

Szewczyk, K. (2007) From the culture of blame to the culture of patients safety. Ethical aspects of medical errors. *Family Medicine and Primary Care Review*: 9: 963–970.

Tate, P. (2007) *The Doctors Communication Handbook (fifth edition)*. Oxford, Radcliffe Publishing.

Taylor, C., Graham, J., Potts, H.W.W., Richards, M.A., and Ramirez, A.J. (2005) Changes in mental health of UK hospital consultants since the mid-1990s. *The Lancet*: 366: 742–744.

Teutsch, C. (2003) Patient-doctor communication. *Medical Clinics of North America*: 87: 1115–45.

Thistlethwaite, J.E., & Jordan, J.J. (1999) Patient-centred consultations: a comparison of student experience and understanding in two clinical environments. *Medical Education*: 33: 678–685.

Thornton, H. (2003) Patients' understanding of risk. *BMJ*: 693–694.

Tomm, K. (1988) Interventive interviewing: Part III. Intending to ask lineal, circular, strategic, or reflexive questions? *Fam Proc*: 27: 1–15.

Travaline, J.M., Ruchinskas, R., and D'Alonzo G.E.Jr. (2005) Patient-physician communication: Why and how. *JAOA*: 105: 13–18.

Trust in People/Trust in Doctors. Ipsos MORI/RCP September 2009 http://www.ipsos-mori.com/Assets/Docs/Polls/poll-trust-in-professions-topline-2009.pdf Accessed 23rd November 2009

Tuckett, D., Boulton, M., Olson, C., and Williams, A. (1985) *Meetings between experts: an approach to sharing ideas in medical consultations*. London, Tavistock.

Turner, J. (2001) Medically unexplained symptoms in secondary care: Consider the possibility of anxiety or depression – or simply distress. *BMJ*: 322: 745–746.

Turton, J. (1998) Importance of information following myocardial infarction: a study of the self-perceived information needs of patients and their spouse/partner compared with the perceptions of nursing staff. *Journal of Advanced Nursing*: 27(4): 770–778.

Van Dalen, J., Kerkhofs, E., Verwijnen, G.M., Knippenberg-van den Berg, B.W., van den Hout, H.A., Scherpbier, A.J.J.A., and van der Vleuten, C.P.M. (2002) Predicting communication skills with a paper-and-pencil test. *Medical Education*: 36: 148–153.

Van Dulmen, S., Sluijs, E., van Kijk, L., de Ridder, D., Heerdink, R., and Bensing, J. (2008) Furthering patient adherence: A position paper of the international expert forum on patient adherence based on an Internet forum discussion. *BMC Health Services Research*: 8: 1472–6963.

References

Vetto, J.T., Elder, N.C., Toffler, W.L., Fields, S.A. (1999) Teaching medical students to give bad news: does formal instruction help? *J Cancer Edu*: 14: 13–17.

Von Fragstein, M., Silverman, J., Cushing, A., Quilligan, S., Salisbury, H., and Wiskin, C. (2008) UK consensus statement on the content of communication curricula in undergraduate medical education. *Med Educ*: 42: 1100–1107.

Van Hemert, A.M., Hengeveld, M.W., Bolk, J.H., Rooijmans, H.G., and Vandenbroucke, J.P. (1993) Psychiatric disorders in relation to medical illness among patients of a general medical out-patient clinic. *Psychol Med*: 23: 167–173.

Waitzkin, H. (1984) Doctor-patient communication. Clinical implications of social scientific research. *JAMA*: 252: 2441–2446.

Waitzkin, H. (1985) Information giving in medical care. *J. Health Soc Behav*: 26: 81–101.

Wass, V. (2005) Ensuring medical students are "fit for purpose". *BMJ*: 331: 791–2.

Wasserman, R.C., & Inui, T.S. (1983) Systematic analysis of clinician-patient interactions: A critique of recent approaches with suggestions for future research. *Medical Care*: 21: 279–293.

Waterman, A., Blades, M., and Spencer, C. (2001) Is a jumper angrier than a tree? *Psychology*: 14: 474–477.

Weiner, S.J., Barnet, B., Cheng, T.L., and Daaleman, T.P. (2005) Processes for effective communication in primary care. *Ann Intern Med*: 142: 709–714.

Weston, W.W., & Brown, J.B. (1989) The importance of patients' beliefs. In: Stewart, M., & Roter, D. editors, *Communicating with Medical Patients*, Beverley Hills, CA, Sage Publications, pp 77–85.

Weston, W.W., & Lipkin, M. Jr. (1989) Doctors learning communication skills: Developmental issues. In: Stewart, M., & Roter, D. editors, *Communicating with Medical Patients*, Beverley Hills, CA, Sage Publications, pp 43–57.

White, J., Levinson, W., and Roter, D. (1994) "Oh by the way...": The closing moments of the medical visit. *J Gen Intern Med*: 9: 24–28.

'Why some doctors are rubbish.' *The Times* (January 23, 2007).

Wikipedia. *Emotional Intelligence*. Online http://en.wikipedia.org/wiki/Emotional_intelligence 5 Oct 2009.

Willard, C., & Luker, K. (2007) Working with the team: Strategies employed by hospital cancer nurse specialists to implement their role. *Journal of Clinical Nursing*: 16: 716–724.

Winefield, H.R., & Chur-Hansen, A. (2000) Evaluating the outcome of communication skill teaching for entry-level medical students: does knowledge of empathy increase? *Medical Education*: 34: 90–94.

Williams, S., Weinman, J., Dale, J., and Newman, S. (1995) Patient expectations: What do primary care patients want from the FP and how far does meeting expectations affect patient satisfaction? *Family Practice*: 12: 193–201.

Williams, S., Weinman, J., and Dale, J. (1998) Doctor-patient communication and patient satisfaction: a review. *Family Practice*: 15: 480–492.

Willis, S.C., Jones, A., and O'Neill, P.A. (2003) Can undergraduate education have an effect on the ways in which pre-registration house officers conceptualise communication? *Medical Education*: 37: 603–608.

Wissow, L.S., Roter, D.L., and Wilson, M.E.H. (1994) Pediatrician interview style and mothers´disclosure of psychosocial issues. *Pediatrics*: 93: 289–295.

Woloshin, S., Schwartz, L.M., and Ellner, A. (2003) Making sense of risk information on the web. *BMJ*: 695–696.

Yedida, M.J., Gillespie, C.C., Kachur, E., Schwartz, M.D., Ockene, J., Chepaitis, A.E., Snyder, C.W., Lazare, A., and Lipkin, M.Jr. (2003) Effect of communications training on medical student performance. *JAMA*: 290: 1157–1165.

Zoppi, K., & Epstein, R.M. (2002) Is communication a skill? Communication behaviors and being in relation. *Family Medicine*: 34: 319–324.

Index

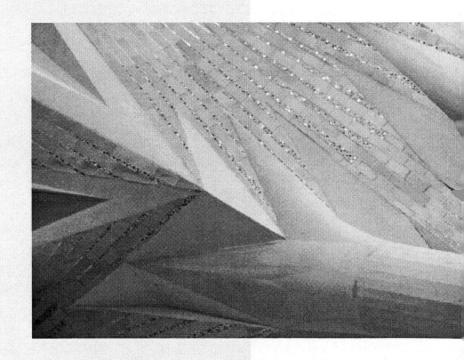

Index

Index

More titles in the Progressing Your Medical Career Series

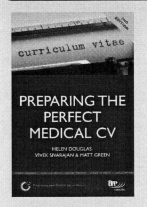

Are you unsure of how to structure your Medical CV? Would you like to know how to ensure you stand out from the crowd?

With competition for medical posts at an all time high it is vital that your Medical CV stands out over your fellow applicants. This comprehensive, unique and easy-to-read guide has been written with this in mind to help prospective medical students, current medical students and doctors of all grades prepare a Medical CV of the highest quality. Whether you are applying to medical school, currently completing your medical degree or a doctor progressing through your career (foundation doctor, specialty trainee in general practice, surgery or medicine, GP career grade or consultant) this guide includes specific guidance for applicants at every level.

This time-saving and detailed guide:

October 2011

Paperback

978-1-445381-62-6

- Explains what selection panels are looking for when reviewing applications at all levels.

- Discusses how to structure your Medical CV to ensure you stand out for the right reasons.

- Explores what information to include (and not to include) in your CV.

- Covers what to consider when maintaining a portfolio at every step of your career, including, for revalidation and relicensing purposes.

- Provides examples of high quality CVs to illustrate the above.

This unique guide will show you how to prepare your CV for every step of your medical career from pre-medical school right through to consultant level and should be a constant companion to ensure you secure your first choice post every time.

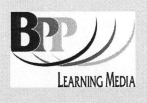

www.bpp.com/health

More titles in the Progressing Your Medical Career Series

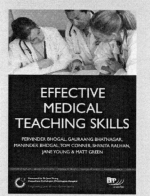

EFFECTIVE MEDICAL TEACHING SKILLS

PERVINDER BHOGAL, GAURAANG BHATNAGAR, MANINDER BHOGAL, TOM CONNER, SHYAITA RALHAN, JANE YOUNG & MATT GREEN

We can all remember a teacher that inspired us, encouraged us and helped us to excel. But what is it that makes a good teacher and are these skills that can be learned and improved?

As doctors and healthcare professionals we are all expected to teach, to a greater or lesser degree, and this carries a great deal of responsibility. We are helping to develop the next generation and it is essential to pass on the knowledge that we have gained during our experience to date.

This book aims to cover the fundamentals of medical education. It has been designed to be a guide for the budding teacher with practical advice, hints, tips and essential points of reflection designed to encourage the reader to think about what they are doing at each step.

October 2011

Paperback

978-1-445379-55-5

By taking the time to read through this book and completing the exercises contained within it you should:

- Understand the needs of the learner

- Understand the skills required to be an effective teacher

- Understand the various different teaching scenarios, from lectures to problem based teaching, and how to use them effectively

- Understand the importance and sources of feedback

- Be aware of assessment techniques, appraisal and revalidation

This book aims to provide you with a foundation in medical education upon which you can build the skills and attributes to become a competent and skilled teacher.

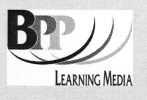

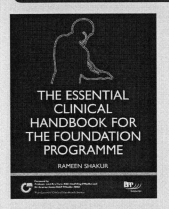
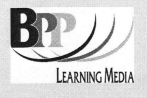

More titles in the Essential Clinical Handbook Series

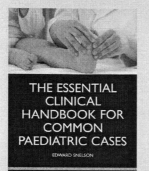

Not sure what to do when faced with a crying baby and demanding parent on the ward? Would you like a definitive guide on how to manage commonly encountered paediatric cases?

This clear and concise clinical handbook has been written to help healthcare professionals approach the initial assessment and management of paediatric cases commonly encountered by Junior Doctors, GPs, GP Specialty Trainee's and allied healthcare professionals. The children who make paediatrics so fun, can also make it more than a little daunting for even the most confident person. This insightful guide has been written based on the author's extensive experience within both a General Practice and hospital setting.

Intended as a practical guide to common paediatric problems it will increase confidence and satisfaction in managing these conditions. Each chapter provides a clear structure for investigating potential paediatric illnesses including clinical and non-clinical advice covering: background, how to assess, pitfalls to avoid, FAQs and what to tell parents. This helpful guide provides :

- A problem/symptom based approach to common paediatric conditions

- An essential guide for any doctor assessing children on the front line

- Provides easy-to-follow and step-by-step guidance on how to approach different paediatric conditions

- Useful both as a textbook and a quick reference guide when needed on the ward

This engaging and easy to use guide will provide you with the knowledge, skills and confidence required to effectively diagnose and manage commonly encountered paediatric cases both within a primary and secondary care setting.

September 2011

Paperback

978-1-445379-60-9

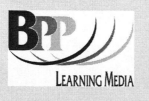

www.bpp.com/health

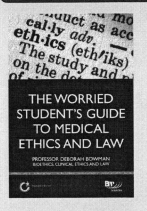
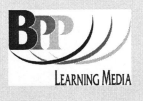